Ace the CSC®!

You Can Do It!

Cardiac Surgery Certification
Study Guide

Nicole Kupchik

MN, RN, CCNS, CCRN-CMC, PCCN-K

Nicole Kupchik Consulting, Inc.
Seattle, WA

Seattle, WA

www.nicolekupchikconsulting.com

This book is dedicated to my mother, Carol.
She passed away January 26, 2019. She was always my biggest
cheerleader and so proud of me. I will love you forever Mom.

Special thanks...

To Carl—what can I say? Book number 6...
your patience with me is beyond astounding. The support &
encouragement you have given me has been incredible.
I owe you one! (Maybe a few actually!)

My many awesome friends—you all know who you are.

Helen Wing—I wouldn't have survived
the past few years without you.

Gina O'Daniel—You always come through with
amazing book covers!

Dr. Elizabeth Bridges—My continual mentor

My friends at Harborview, Swedish, Overlake & Evergreen
who have always encouraged me over the years!

And the THOUSANDS of nurses who attended my classes,
gave constructive feedback and took the exams!
You are all an inspiration to me!

The encouragement you all have given me is immeasurable
and completely appreciated!

Unless we are making
progress in our nursing
every year, every month, every week,
take my word for it,
we are going back.

—Florence Nightingale (May 1872)

Contents

Contents

A note of encouragement from Nicole

Congratulations on taking steps to becoming certified and obtaining the CSC® subspecialty certification!

In 2002, I passed the CCRN® for the first time. I am going to let you in on a little secret. I was eligible to sit the exam in 1994. I attended three certification review courses before taking the exam. Why? I lacked confidence and was so afraid of failing. I finally got up the courage in 2002 and aced it!

I can distinctly remember walking out of the testing site questioning myself and why I waited so long to take it. I had so much self-doubt. It was a little crazy, because clinically, I knew my stuff. A couple years later I started teaching sections of the exam at Harborview and in 2006 started co-teaching the prep courses nationally.

Who would think someone could go from having a complete lack of confidence to teaching the courses a few years later?! Mental mindset is everything. I want you to tell yourself every day that you can do this!!!

I often hear nurses say "becoming certified doesn't make you a better nurse". I completely disagree with statements like that. The journey you will take in preparing to become certified increases your knowledge to better advocate and care for your patients. I truly believe every nurse should be certified in their specialty.

The CSC® exam was a long-term professional goal. Much of my career was dedicated to the care of post-operative Cardiac Surgery patients. It was with this population I mastered hemodynamics. Again, I was fearful to sit the exam, but did and aced it. Being prepared is the key to becoming certified. I was so proud to obtain this certification.

I was inspired to publish this book by nurses who attended my review courses. Many of the study books available are overwhelming & contain too much information. My goal is always to break down disease states into digestible pieces so you can learn & understand the content! I did this for the CCRN® & PCCN®. Now I want to offer a review book for the CSC®.

My biggest piece of advice to you in studying is, of course to understand different conditions, but do as many practice test questions as possible. Read the rationales for questions you get right & those you miss. I believe that is the key to success.

Thank you to the following contributors:

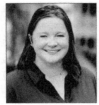

Michelle A. Dedeo DNP, RN, CNS, ACCNS-AG, CCRN

Michelle received her Bachelors of Science in Nursing from the University of Wisconsin Madison and her Masters in Nursing and Doctorate in Nursing Practice from the University of Washington. She works for Legacy Health and teaches for Linfield College, both in Portland, OR.

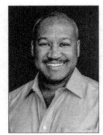

James "Charlie" Edwards MSN-Ed, RN, CCRN-K, CEN

Charlie earned a Bachelor of Science in Nursing from the University of Phoenix and a Master of Science in Nursing Education from Western Governors University. He has been a nurse for over 27 years and is currently the Director of Nursing Professional Practice / Education Services at Desert Regional Medical Center in Palm Springs, California.

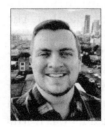

Joel Green MSN, RN, CCRN-CMC, CSC

Joel Green lives in Seattle, Washington, and is currently working in the Medical Cardiac ICU at a Level 1 Trauma Center. He has a Master's Degree in Nursing Education and has been a Registered Nurse for over 16 years. He has worked in telemetry, critical care, post anesthesia care, and for medical device companies as an educator.

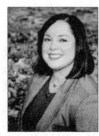

Kimberly Kelly MSN, RN, CCRN-CSC

Kimberly Kelly has been a registered nurse, specializing in critical care and open-heart recovery for over 13 years. She graduated with her BSN in 2006 from Ferris State University, and in 2018 obtained an MSN from Western Governors University. Originally from Michigan, she moved to Oregon in 2008, where she started getting involved in her local AACN chapter. For years, Kimberly has been very involved in the Greater Portland Chapter of AACN. She has taken on numerous board positions, from chairing and executing the GPC-AACN Critical Care Fall Symposium, to President of the chapter. Kimberly recently left bedside nursing to pursue another avenue of nursing. She is currently a Clinical Consultant for Cheetah Medical.

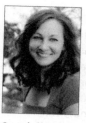

Kristin Nathan BSN, RN, CCRN

Kristin Nathan has been a registered nurse, specializing in critical care, post open heart recovery and resuscitation, for over 20 years. She graduated with her BSN in 1995 from The Ohio State University. She is currently pursuing her Masters in Nursing Education from Oregon Health & Sciences University and works as a Nursing Education and Simulation Specialist at Legacy Emanuel Medical Center in Portland, Oregon.

Kristin has worked as a clinical adjunct faculty at Linfield Good Samaritan School of Nursing and was recently a clinical unit educator for 5 years in a cardiovascular ICU. She has developed an open-heart training program and protocols related to care management with post open heart recovery and is certified in cardiac surgery advanced life support. Kristin has spoken nationally promoting CCRN certification and has collaborated with the Greater Portland Chapter of AACN speaking on hemodynamics for their statewide critical care nursing consortium.

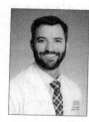

Todd D. Ray DNP, ARNP, ACNP, RN

Todd received his Bachelors of Science in Zoology from the University of Idaho and his Bachelors of Science in Nursing from Lewis-Clark State College. He completed his Masters in Nursing and Doctorate in Nursing Practice from the University of Washington. He currently works at the University of Washington as a Teaching Associate for the Division of Cardiology and as an Associate Professor for the University of Washington School of Nursing. In his spare time Todd plays bagpipes for the Keith Highlanders Pipe Band, and volunteers at Carepoint (a free health care clinic) in the Snoqualmie valley and is an avid fly fisherman. Todd resides in Snoqualmie, Washington, with is fiancé Jody, and children Kaitlin, Grace and Julian.

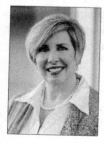

Theresa L. Reed BSN, RN, CCRN-CSC

Theresa has her Bachelors of Science in Nursing and has been a Critical Care/Cardiovascular Surgery RN for 35 years. Her former position was a Cardiovascular Care coordinator at CHI Harrison Medical Center until June 2017 with educational responsibilities for ICU, PCU and OR Open Heart Staff and Cath Lab. She now resides in Snohomish, Washington.

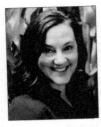

Amy Stafford MN, RN, CCNS, CCRN

Amy received her Bachelors of Science in Nursing from Saint Joseph's College of Maine and her Masters in Nursing from the University of Washington. She has over 20 years of experience working in critical care in various capacities. She currently works as the Manager of Nursing Academic Affairs at Maine Medical Center in Portland, ME.

Reviewers

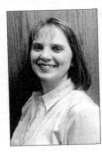

Nancy Hammond MSN, RN, CCRN, TCRN

Nancy has been a nurse taking care of critically ill patients for 18 years. Graduating with her Bachelors of Science in Nursing from Maryville University in 2000, Nancy started her nursing career on a Cardiac Telemetry unit and quickly realized she wanted to take care of higher acuity patients. In 2004 Nancy began working in a combined Medical/Cardiac/Neurological ICU. As an integral member of the ICU team, Nancy developed and implemented a mentoring program for ICU new hires significantly decreasing turnover and it was adopted in multiple SSM facilities. In 2008 Nancy accepted a leadership role as a charge nurse managing the ICU. During this time Nancy realized her passion for precepting, mentoring and educating all nurses. In 2010, Nancy obtained a Master's degree in Nursing Education from Webster University in St. Louis which opened doors for opportunities as a respected educator.

In 2014, Nancy accepted the role of Clinical Educator at SSM Health DePaul Hospital. She continues to pursue her passion in nursing education, teaching all topics related to the care of the critically ill patient. Nancy enjoys teaching others and sharing her passion, knowing this directly impacts the quality of patient care.

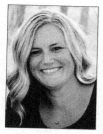

Meghan Holland MSN, RN, CCRN, CNML

Meghan Holland is a Senior Nurse Manager at Bayhealth Medical Center in Dover, Delaware. She graduated from the University of Delaware in 2010 with a MSN with a focus as an adult Clinical Nurse Specialist. She has been practicing in critical care for a total 15 years, 14 of which have been in Cardiovascular Surgery. She has helped implement programs for the CVSICU team, such as Impella, ECMO and is certified in both critical care and nursing leadership. She was an AONE Nurse Manager Fellow in 2014.

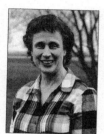

Mary Patricia Logan MSN, RN, CCRN-K, TCRN

Pat received her diploma from St. Luke's Hospital School of Nursing in St. Louis, Missouri in 1987. She earned her Bachelor and Master of Science in Nursing from Webster University in 1991 and 2005, respectively. She has held adjunct faculty positions at Webster University and Lindenwood University and has led review courses through Kaplan University. Pat has spent the last 32 years as a critical care nurse and is currently a Clinical Educator for Critical Care at SSM Health DePaul Hospital in St. Louis, Missouri.

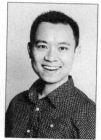

Tao Zheng MN, RN, CCRN-CSC-CMC, CHFN, PCCN

Tao lives in Chicago, Illinois. He received his Bachelor of Science in Nursing from Olympic College and his Masters in Nursing Education from University of Washington. Tao currently works as a Clinical Nurse Educator (cardiovascular specialty) in the Center for Nursing Professional Practice and Research at the University of Chicago Medicine.

Tao has worked as an adjunct faculty in multiple nursing schools. Clinically, he has worked in surgical telemetry, cardiothoracic intensive care unit, and cardiac cath lab.

You Can Do It!

About the Cardiac Surgery–CSC® Subspecialty Certification Exam

The CSC® is administered by the American Association of Critical Care Nurses (AACN). Their website information can be found at: www.aacn.org

Qualifications to sit the exam:

- Hold a current unencumbered nursing license

- A current nursing certification to attach
  - Must be nationally accredited
  - Example: CCRN, PCCN, CCNS

- Practice as RN or APRN for 1,750 hours direct care of adult patients; 875 care of acutely/critically ill adult cardiac surgery **OR**

- RN or APRN with 5 years experience, minimum of 2,000 hours, 144 in most recent year.

- If you have any questions about eligibility, please contact AACN – they are super helpful!

The online application has a fast turnaround time and requests demographic information including your nursing license number. In addition, you will need to provide the name and contact information of a colleague or manager who can verify your eligibility. Once your application has been processed and you are deemed eligible, you will receive an email from AACN. Next, a company called PSI will email instructions to schedule your exam. You have 90 days to schedule and sit your exam. (Note: during the pandemic, the test window was extended to 180 days). Easy peasy!

The CSC® exam consists of 90 questions. Fifteen questions will not count toward your final score. They are used for statistical data for future exams. It's kind of a bummer you don't know which questions don't count! The advice I ALWAYS give nurses—if you come across a question that you have NO idea the answer, tell yourself it's a question that doesn't count, don't psych yourself out if you don't know the answer. There will be some questions you just may not know!

Exam questions are written at the application & analysis levels based on Synergy model of care; meaning they aren't super basic questions. They want to know you understand how to take care of patients and what to anticipate in treatment. On that same thought, they also aren't trying to trick you. Each question will have 4 answer choices and only one is the correct answer.

You will have 2 hours to complete the exam. The most recent published pass rate for the CSC® exam is 72.6%. The passing "cut score" is 55 correct out of 75. Translated—you have to get about 73% correct to pass. The way they score is a little more complicated than a straight 73%, but I'm not completely sure exactly how that's calculated. You can easily do this, but you need to be prepared.

Cardiac Surgery Certification (CSC) Test Plan

Applies to exams taken on or after January 31, 2022.

I. PROCEDURES (11%)

A. Cardiovascular

1. Coronary artery bypass surgery (CABG) with cardiopulmonary bypass
2. Coronary artery bypass surgery (CABG) without cardiopulmonary bypass
3. Cox maze and modified maze procedure
4. Minimally invasive cardiac surgery
5. Pericardial window
6. Repair of non-congenital heart defects (e.g., left-ventricular aneurysm, VSD post MI)
7. Surgical valve repair or replacement
8. Transcatheter valve replacement (e.g., TAVR)

B. Thoracic

1. Endovascular repair of the aorta
2. Open repair of thoracic aortic aneurysm or dissection

II. COMPLICATIONS (33%)

A. Cardiovascular

1. Cardiogenic shock
2. Hypotension and hypertension
3. Hypovolemia and hypervolemia
4. Bleeding
5. Myocardial infarction
6. Myocardial stunning
7. Open chest from the operating room
8. Pericarditis
9. Dysrhythmias
10. Right heart failure
11. Cardiac tamponade
12. Vascular complications (e.g., compartment syndrome, retroperitoneal bleeding)

B. Respiratory

1. Acute respiratory failure
2. Acute respiratory distress syndrome (ARDS)
3. Transfusion related acute lung injury (TRALI)
4. Transfusion associated circulatory overload (TACO)
5. Pleural space abnormalities (e.g., pneumothorax)
6. Air-leak syndromes (e.g., pneumopericardium, pneumomediastinum)
7. Aspiration
8. Atelectasis
9. Pleural effusion
10. Prolonged mechanical ventilation
11. Pulmonary hypertension

C. Endocrine

1. Hyperglycemia and hypoglycemia

D. Hematology / Immunology

1. Protamine reactions
2. Coagulopathies
3. Anemia
4. Heparin-induced thrombocytopenia (HIT)

E. Neurology

1. Postoperative impaired cognition
2. Cerebrovascular accident (stroke)
3. Lower limb deficits (e.g., spinal cord ischemia, paralysis)
4. Delirium

F. Gastrointestinal

1. Ischemic bowel

G. Renal

1. Acute kidney injury
2. Electrolyte imbalances

H. Multisystem

1. Multisystem organ dysfunction syndrome (MODS)
2. Chronic pain
3. Acute pain
4. Acid-base imbalances
5. Malignant hyperthermia

I. Behavioral / Psychosocial

1. Preexisting behavioral health disorder (e.g., anxiety, PTSD)
2. Substance use and withdrawal

III. THERAPEUTIC INTERVENTIONS (43%)

A. Cardiovascular

1. Fluid volume management specific to cardiac surgery
2. Defibrillation and cardioversion
3. Emergent resternotomy
4. Cardiac surgery advanced life support (CALS)
5. Temporary pacing
6. Intra-aortic balloon pump
7. Short-term ventricular assist devices (VADs)
8. Extracorporeal membrane oxygenation (ECMO)
9. Pericardial and mediastinal drain

B. Pharmacology

1. Platelet inhibitors
2. Thrombolytics
3. Anticoagulants
4. Vasoactive agents
5. Antidysrhythmics
6. Inotropes
7. Diuretics
8. Beta-blockers
9. Statins
10. Pharmacologic agents for controlling bleeding
    (e.g., desmopressin acetate, factor VII, antifibrinolytics)
11. Pulmonary vasodilators
12. Sedation
13. Neuromuscular blockade

C. Respiratory

1. Pleural chest tubes and drains
2. Invasive and non-invasive mechanical ventilation
3. Oxygen therapy delivery devices
4. Post-extubation care

D. Endocrine

1. Glycemic control

E. Hematology and Immunology

1. Blood and blood products

F. Neurology

1. Lumbar drain
2. Pain management

G. Renal

1. Renal replacement therapy (e.g., hemodialysis, CRRT)

H. Standards of Care

1. Deep vein thrombosis (DVT) prophylaxis
2. Early mobility protocols
3. Gastrointestinal (GI) prophylaxis
4. Surgical site protocols
5. Recovery from anesthesia
6. Rewarming from hypothermia
7. Pneumonia prevention

IV. MONITORING AND DIAGNOSTICS (13%)

A. Cardiovascular

1. Hemodynamic monitoring
2. Echocardiography
3. Electrocardiography (ECG)
4. Laboratory testing

B. Respiratory

1. Arterial blood gas (ABG)
2. Mixed venous gas
3. Pulse oximetry
4. Capnography
5. Radiography

C. Neurology

1. Bispectral index monitoring (BIS)
2. Cerebral oximetry monitoring
3. Train-of-four (TOF)

Order of content does not necessarily reflect importance.

You Can Do It!

Chapter 1

Cardiac Basics

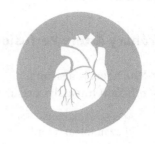

Topics covered in this chapter include:

- ▶ Coronary artery perfusion
- ▶ Basic Hemodynamic concepts
- ▶ Heart sounds
- ▶ Heart valves

Cardiac Basics

Coronary Artery Perfusion

» The heart is a strong, efficient muscular organ

* At rest, it extracts 70% of available oxygen!

» Both the right & left **coronary arteries** arise at the base of the aorta (Sinus of Valsalva); immediately above the aortic valve

» Two main coronary arteries: Right & left

» Coronary arteries are perfused during...?

* DIASTOLE!

* This is why tachycardia is so challenging in heart failure & cardiovascular disease!

* Tachycardia = ↓ perfusion time & diastolic filling time

» Coronary perfusion pressure (CPP) =

* Diastolic BP minus left ventricular end diastolic pressure (LVEDP)

* Normal CPP = > 40 mm Hg

» Atrial contraction (atrial kick) contributes about 20 – 25% of cardiac output

* SO, when patients go into atrial fibrillation, they lose that **atrial kick**!

* In low EF states/heart failure, they may not tolerate Afib so well!

Coronary Circulation

1) The RIGHT Coronary Artery (RCA) perfuses the:

» ***Inferior Wall**

» Right atrium

» SA Node (> 50% of population)

» AV Node

» Right ventricle

» Posterior portion of the septum

» Posterior wall in ~ 90% of the population

RCA branches = Acute marginal & posterior descending

2) The **Left Main artery** perfuses the left side of the heart

Think *MAJOR PUMP!*

Nickname (if vessel is occluded) = WIDOW MAKER!!!

» Left main occlusion
= bad prognosis

The **Left Main Artery** bifurcates into the:

» Left Anterior Descending
(LAD) Artery &

» Left Circumflex Artery

FYI – In CABG, usually don't directly graft the left main (anatomically unable)

The **Left Anterior Descending (LAD)** perfuses the:

» ***Septal & Anterior Wall**

» Front & apex of left ventricle

• 50% of blood flow to the LV

» Most of the interventricular
septum

» Anterior papillary muscle

» Most of the left & right
bundle branches

» Bundle of His

» *The LAD is the most
commonly occluded artery

The **Left Circumflex** perfuses the:

» ***Lateral Wall**

» Left atrium

» Back of left ventricle

» Posterior wall in ~ 10%
of the population

Some people (~ 20% of the population) have a **Ramus artery** (tertiary left main)

» Runs along the left ventricle
between the LAD & circumflex

Basic Hemodynamic Concepts

Preload

The initial stretching of the myocardium prior to contraction; therefore, it is related to the sarcomere length at the end of diastole.

» Equated to volume status (with caution!)

» High preload = fluid overload (But not always clinically true!)

» Low preload = fluid deficit (again, not always true!)

» Pulmonary Artery Catheter measurement on the:

- Right side of the heart as the central venous pressure "CVP" or right atrial pressure "RAP"

- Left side of the heart as the pulmonary artery occlusive pressure or "PAOP" or "wedge" pressure

Afterload

» The **resistance** the ventricles have to overcome to eject blood

- Systemic vascular resistance (SVR) = the resistance the left ventricle has to overcome to eject

- Peripheral vascular resistance (PVR) = the resistance the right ventricle has to overcome to eject

» High afterload = **Vasoconstriction**

» Low afterload = **Vasodilation**

Heart Sounds

Valvular auscultation points:

» Aortic valve: Right sternal border, 2nd ICS

» Pulmonic valve: Left sternal border, 2nd ICS

» Tricuspid valve: Left sternal border, 4 - 5th ICS

» Mitral valve: Mid-clavicular line, 5th ICS

Normal Heart Sounds

» S_1: closure of the mitral & tricuspid valves

- Loudest over mitral area
- Systole
- 1/3 of the cardiac cycle
- "LUB"

» S_2: closure of pulmonic & aortic valve

- Loudest over aortic area, 2nd ICS
- Diastole
- 2/3 of the cardiac cycle
- "DUB"

Extra Heart Sounds

» S_3: Ventricular Gallop

- Auscultated in fluid overload; when preload is elevated
- Normal in kids, high cardiac output, 3rd trimester of pregnancy
- Listen over apex area
- "Ken-tuck-y" or "I Believe" cadence

» S_4: Atrial gallop (pre-systolic)

- Sound caused by vibration of atria ejecting into non-compliant ventricles
- Auscultated during ischemia (increased resistance to ventricular filling)
- Other causes: Ischemia, HTN, pulmonary stenosis, CAD, Aortic stenosis, left ventricular hypertrophy
- Listen over tricuspid or mitral area
- "Ten-ne-see" or "Believe-me" cadence

» **Split Heart Sounds**

- When one valve closes later than the other
  ▷ **best heard during *inspiration***
- Split S_1 - Mitral closes before tricuspid valve
  ▷ RBBB, PVCs, ventricular paced rhythms
- Split S_2 - Aortic closes before pulmonic valve.
  ▷ Overfilled right ventricle
  ▷ Atrial septal defect (ASD)

Heart Valves

Atrioventricular (A-V) Valves:

» Mitral (on the left) & Tricuspid (on the right) and are:

- Open during - DIASTOLE!

- Closed during - SYSTOLE!

» The papillary muscle & chordae tendineae control the opening & closing of the AV valves with pressure changes

- Prevent the inversion/prolapse of the AV valves during systole

Semilunar Valves

» Aortic (on the left) & Pulmonic (on the right) and are:

- Open during - SYSTOLE!

- Closed during - DIASTOLE!

You Can Do It!

Cardiac Medications

Class	Examples	Indications	Effects	Monitor for:	Watch out!
ACE Inhibitors	"prils" —take a "chill-pril"! Class I: Captopril Class II: Enalapril (Vasotec) Ramipril (Altace) Benazepril (Lotensin) Class III: Lisinopril	-CHF/Systolic failure -AMI (EF < 40%) -Anterior wall MI -HTN -Diabetic renal nephropathy	-Vasodilation ↓ preload & afterload -Prevention of myocardial remodeling -Reduce progress of diabetic nephropathy	↓ BP ↑ K⁺ levels ↑ Creatinine	Hypotension Cough Hyperkalemia Angioedema Renal function
Beta Blockers	"olols" **Cardio-selective (blocks B₁):** * Bisoprolol, *Metoprolol SR, Atenolol, Esmolol (IV), Acebutolol, Nebivolol (Bystolic) **Alpha & Beta Blocking:** Labetalol, *Carvedilol (Coreg) **Non-selective (blocks B₁ & B₂):** Propranolol (Inderal), Timolol, Nadolol (Corgard), Sotalol * used in heart failure	-Secondary prevention of MI (only metoprolol tartrate or carvedilol) -Cardiac arrhythmias -Angina -Afib -CHF/Systolic failure -HTN	BB = **B**lock the heart **B**reaks on the heart (↓HR) -↓ HR, BP -Negative inotrope, however, decreases myocardial workload -↓ preload -Block endogenous epi & norepi; "stress catecholamine" -↓ morbidity & mortality in HF -↓ arrhythmias	↓ HR ↓ BP AV Blocks Heart failure	Bradycardia Hypotension Signs of shock Bronchospasm; Avoid in asthma! Heart block Avoid with cocaine use **Overdose reversal:** Glucagon
Angiotension Receptor Blockers (ARBs)	"sartans" Valsartan, Losartan, Candesartan, Olmesartan, Telmisartan	-HTN -CHF/Systolic failure -Diabetic renal nephropathy -Intolerance of ACE Inhibitors	-Vasodilation -Decreases preload & afterload -Reduces secretion of vasopressin	↓ BP ↑ K⁺ levels ↑ Creatinine	Dizziness Headache Hyperkalemia Caution: MI

Aldosterone Blockers	Spironolactone (Aldactone), Eplerenone (Inspra)	Adjunctive therapy in heart failure	-Diuresis -Blocks Na+ reabsorption -↓ preload & afterload -In combo with other diuretics, ↓ cardiac workload -K+ sparing diuretic	↑ K+ levels	Hyperkalemia—especially when used with ACE Inhibitors or ARBs
Calcium Channel Blockers (CCBs)	"dipines" used for BP reduction! **Dihydropyridines:** (little effect on contractility or heart rate) Amlodipine, nimodipine, nicardipine (IV), Clevidipine (IV), Nifedipine, Felodipine **Benzothiazepine class:** Diltiazem (Cardizem) - HR control **Phenylalkylamine class:** Verapamil (Calan) - HR control	-HTN -Reduce HR -SVT -Afib/flutter -Angina—Prinzmetal's (vasospasm) -Hypertrophic CM -Prevent cerebral artery vasospasm (nimodipine)	-Arterial vasodilation, ↓ afterload -↓ the force of myocardial contraction -Negative chronotrope -Negative inotrope	↓ HR ↓ BP	Heart block Bradycardia Reflexive tachycardia Caution when used with BB **Overdose:** Calcium Chloride & Atropine
Nitrates	Nitroglycerin Isosorbide dinitrate (Isordil) Isosorbide mononitrate (Imdur)	-Angina -Heart failure	-Vasodilation -Venodilation	↓ BP Headaches	Hypotension
Hydrazinophthalazine	Hydralazine *Usually prescribed in combo with isosorbide tinitrate, a BB & diuretic in heart failure	-Heart failure -HTN	-Vasodilator -↓ afterload	↓ BP Headaches	Reflexive tachycardia MI/angina

Definitions:
Inotrope—has an effect on contractility, positive inotrope improves contractility, negative inotrope decreases contractility.
Chronotrope—has an effect on heart rate, positive chronotrope increases the heart rate, negative chronotrope decreases the heart rate.

Chapter 2

Hemodynamic Monitoring

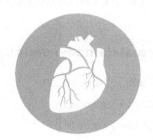

Topics covered in this chapter include:

- ▶ Normal Hemodynamic values
- ▶ Hemodynamic concepts
  - Mixed venous monitoring (ScvO$_2$ & SvO$_2$)
- ▶ Pulmonary Artery Catheter (PAC)
  - Central venous pressure monitoring (without pulmonary artery catheter)
  - Cardiogenic Shock
  - LV & RV Failure
- ▶ Shock Hemodynamics
- ▶ Vasopressors & positive inotropes
  - Vasopressor extravasations
- ▶ Vasodilators

Normal Hemodynamic Values

Normal Hemodynamic Values (Know this!!!)

Cardiac Output (C.O.)	4 – 8 L/min
Cardiac Index (C.I.)	2.5 – 4 L/min/m²
Stroke volume (S.V.)	50 – 100 mL/beat
Stroke volume index (S.V.I.)	35 – 60 ml/beat/m²
Right ventricular stroke work index (RVSWI)	5 – 10 g/m²/beat
Left ventricular stroke work index (LVSWI)	50 – 62 g/m²/beat
SvO$_2$	60 – 75%
ScvO$_2$	> 70% (70 – 85%)
Pulmonary artery pressure	25/10 mm Hg
PAOP	8 – 12 mm Hg
RAP/CVP	2 – 6 mm Hg
SVR	900 - 1400 dynes/sec/cm^{-5}
SVRI	1970 – 2390 dynes/sec/cm^{-5}/m²
PVR	90 - 250 dynes/sec/cm^{-5}

An easy way to remember Intra-Cardiac pressures:

Nickel - Dime - Quarter - Dollar!!!
Because we can ALL relate to $$$!!!

A normal RAP/CVP is about a **nickel**

A normal PAOP is about a **dime**

A normal PAP is about a **quarter** over a **dime**

A normal LV pressure (systolic BP) is about a **dollar**!

You have to know norms! We are so used to looking at abnormal numbers, we forget what norms are! (OR, maybe you rarely see PA catheters...the struggle is real!)

Hemodynamic Concepts

Cardiac output (C.O.):

» Amount of blood ejected by the ventricles per minute

» C.O. = Heart rate (HR) x Stroke volume (SV)

- Normal C.O. = 4 - 8 L/min

- Normal Cardiac Index (C.I.) = 2.5 – 4.0 L/min/m²

- Cardiac index = C.O. ÷ Body Surface Area (BSA)

» C.O. may be normal if the patient is tachycardic with lower SV

- In low output states, patients compensate with tachycardia

» Can be measured:

- Pulmonary artery catheter

- Echocardiogram

- Indirectly via functional hemodynamics

- Non-invasive methods (Bioreactance, continuous digit CO)

- Fick equation (gold standard calculation)

Stroke volume (SV):

» The amount of blood ejected from the ventricles with each beat/contraction

» SV = CO ÷ HR x 1000

- Normal is 50 - 100 mL/beat

- Normal stroke volume index (SVI) = 35 – 60 ml/beat/m²

» SV = End diastolic volume (EDV) – End systolic volume (ESV)

- Typical EDV = 120 ml
  ▷ Amount of blood in the heart at the end of diastole/filling

- Typical ESV = 50 ml
  ▷ Amount of blood in the ventricles at the end of systole/ejection

» Three measures contribute to SV:

- Preload
  ▷ Myocardial fiber length at the end of diastole

- Afterload
  ▷ Resistance the heart has to eject against during systole

- Contractility
  ▷ Strength of myofibril contraction

Preload

» Defined as the stretching of cardiac myocytes prior to ejection

» Volume concept, measured as pressure

» Indirectly measured on the <u>right side</u>:

- Right Atrial Pressure (RAP)
- Central Venous Pressure (CVP)
- Normal 2 – 6 mm Hg
- Estimate of right ventricular end-diastolic pressure (RVEDP)

» End diastole volume or venous return

» Volume of blood filling the ventricle during diastole

» Indirectly measured on the <u>left side</u>:

- Pulmonary Artery Occlusive Pressure (PAOP)
- Normal 8 – 12 mm Hg
- Reflective of left atrial pressure
- PAOP is always lower than the PA diastolic
- Estimate of left ventricular end-diastolic pressure (LVEDP)

Note: The CVP & PAOP are POOR predictors of fluid responsiveness!

Conditions causing an <u>increase</u> in <u>preload</u>:

» Left ventricular heart failure (+/- CVP & ↑PAOP)

» Hypervolemia (+/- CVP & ↑PAOP)

» Pulmonary edema (↑PAOP)

» Cardiogenic shock (+/- CVP & ↑PAOP)

» RV failure (↑CVP with normal PAOP)

- Will likely see LOW LV preload!

» Ventricular septal defect (VSD)

» Pulmonary hypertension (↑CVP, PAP)

» Tricuspid stenosis (↑CVP)

» Mitral stenosis (↑PAOP)

» Pericardial Tamponade (↑CVP & PAOP because heart is compressed)

» Increasing PEEP on the ventilator

- Increased intrathoracic chest pressure
- Also decreases, see below

» IV fluids (at least that's usually the goal)

Treatment of increased preload:

» It depends, but diuresis, vasodilators, +inotrope like Milrinone, decrease the PEEP

Conditions causing a <u>decrease</u> in <u>preload</u>:

» Hypovolemia for whatever reason

» Bleeding

» Veno/vasodilation

- Inflammatory response from cardiopulmonary bypass

» After the administration of Morphine, NTG or beta blockers!

» Decreased venous return

- Increased intravascular pressure
- Hypovolemic
- Will see pulse pressure or stroke volume variability

» Increasing PEEP on the ventilator

- Decreased venous return

Treatment of decreased preload:

» It depends, but volume, back off the PEEP, decrease vasodilator dosing

Afterload (Systemic Vascular Resistance)

» Defined as the pressure or resistance the ventricles must overcome to eject blood

» Pulmonary vascular resistance (PVR)

- Normal 90 - 250 dynes/sec/cm^{-5}
- Formula = $\dfrac{(PAM - PAOP) \times 80}{CO}$

- Elevated with:
  ▷ Cardiopulmonary Bypass (CPB)
  ▷ Mechanical Ventilation
  ▷ Acidosis, Hypoxia
  ▷ ARDS
  ▷ *All of these can lead to RV dysfunction!
  ▷ Monitor for rising CVP

» Systemic vascular resistance (SVR)

- Normal 900 - 1400 dynes/sec/cm^{-5}
- Formula = $\dfrac{(MAP - CVP) \times 80}{CO}$

Conditions causing an <u>increase</u> in <u>afterload</u>:

» Cardiogenic shock

» Hypovolemia/shock

» Bleeding

» Heart failure

» Cardiac tamponade

» Use of catecholamine vasopressors (i.e. epinephrine, norepinephrine)

» Hypothermia

» HTN

Think vasoconstriction!

Treatment of increased afterload:

» It depends, but treat the underlying cause

» Consider: vasodilators (Nipride, Nitroglycerin, Nicardipine, Clevidipine)

Conditions causing a <u>decrease</u> in <u>afterload</u>:

» Vasoplegic shock (coming off bypass!)

» Prolonged CPB – Inflammatory (SIRS) response

» ACE-Inhibitor use prior to surgery

» Hyperthermia

» Anaphylaxis – Concerns with Protamine!

» Vasodilators (i.e. Nitroglycerin, Nipride, although usually intended effect ☺)

» Septic shock (Hyperdynamic stage)

» Spinal/neurogenic shock

Think vasodilation!

Treatment of decreased afterload:

» Vasopressors (NE, Epi,
Vasopressin, Phenylephrine,
Dopamine, Giapreza,
Methylene Blue)

Contractility

» Force of ventricular ejection

» Difficult to measure

» Influenced by changes in
preload & afterload

» "Inotrope" +/-

 • + inotropes will increase
   contractility (i.e. Dobutamine,
   Milrinone, Epi)

 • – inotropes will decrease
   contractility (i.e. beta blockers,
   some calcium channel blockers)

Other factors affecting contractility:

» STEMI/myocardial ischemia

» Myocardial stunning post CPB

» Inadequate stretch

 • Hypovolemia, bleeding

» ↑ Resistance (increased
SVR/afterload)

» ↑ H^+ (acidosis), ↑ CO_2

» Severe hypoxia

» Anesthetics (negative inotropy)

» Sepsis (can cause
hyperdynamic CO)

Treatment – reverse underlying metabolic conditions

» Vasodilate if d/t ↑ SVR

» + inotrope (Dobutamine,
Milrinone, Epi)

» Mechanical assistance
(IABP, Impella, VAD)

SvO$_2$

» True mixed venous O$_2$ saturation

» Measures relationship between oxygen delivery & consumption

  • Early warning of ↓ CO

  • Big goal post-op is to maintain the DO$_2$/VO$_2$ balance!

  • Normal SvO$_2$ 60 – 75%

  • Measured with a pulmonary artery catheter

» Normal oxygen extraction ratio (O$_2$ER) = 25 – 30%

» In other words, we normally extract 25 – 30% of oxygen to the tissues & 70 – 75% comes back to the heart and is measured via SvO$_2$ or ScvO$_2$

» ScvO$_2$ 70% - 85%

  • Surrogate of mixed venous – central venous

  • Measurement from the SVC

  • Runs about 5 – 8% higher than SvO$_2$

  • Trends with SvO$_2$

  • If you cannot continuously monitor:

    ▷ Draw sample from distal tip of TLC/PICC (thorax) that is positioned in the Superior Vena Cava

If SvO$_2$ or ScvO$_2$ is low, first ask yourself if it is a delivery or consumption problem, or BOTH?!

» DO$_2$ (O$_2$ delivery) is affected by 3 physiologic parameters:

  • "The Pump"

    ▷ Is the cardiac output adequate?

  • "The Lungs"

    ▷ Is the oxygenation adequate? Excessive metabolic demands?

  • "The Hemoglobin"

    ▷ Is there adequate O$_2$ carrying capacity?

» VO$_2$ (↑ O$_2$ consumption) is affected by:

  • Increased work of breathing

  • Shivering

  • Fever

  • Infection

  • Agitation

  • Turning

  • Nursing care

  • Environment

The Pulmonary Artery Catheter (PAC)

a.k.a. "Swan-Ganz" catheter

Contraindications to use of a PA Catheter:

» Tricuspid or pulmonic prosthetic valve

» Right heart mass (thrombus or tumor)

» Tricuspid or pulmonic valve endocarditis

» Left BBB

Direct measurements from PAC:

» Right atrial pressure (RAP/CVP)

» Pulmonary artery pressures (PAS/PAD)

» Pulmonary artery occlusive pressure (PAOP)

» C.O.

» SvO_2

Calculated measurements:

» SV/SVI

» C.I.

» SVR/SVRI

» PVR

» DO_2

In other words, everything else is just algebra!

Guidelines for PAC use:

» **Level at the phlebostatic axis**

• 4th ICS & ½ AP diameter (level of left atrium)

• Eliminates effects of hydrostatic forces on the observed hemodynamic

• Ensure air-fluid interface of the transducer is leveled before zeroing &/or obtaining pressure readings

» **0 - 60° HOB elevation**

» **Dynamic response testing (a.k.a square wave test)**

- Fast flush – should see 1 – 3 oscillatory waves following flush

- Optimal test ensures the line is reliable

» **Overdamped waveform:**

- Sluggish, artificially rounded & blunted appearance

- SBP erroneously low; DBP erroneously high

- Causes: large air bubbles in system, compliant tubing, loose/open connections, and low fluid level in flush bag

» **Underdamped waveform:**

- Over responsive, exaggerated, artificially spiked waveform

- SBP erroneously high; DBP erroneously low

- Causes: small air bubbles, too long of tubing, defective transducer

Rules for measuring CVP & PAOP waveforms:

» Measure at end-expiration

» Measure the mean of the a – c wave

» Ensure transducer is leveled at the Phlebostatic axis

» Ensure line is reliable (dynamic response test) – for all lines including arterial

RAP/CVP & PAOP waveforms consist of:

» a wave - upstroke of atrial systole

- Produced after atrial depolarization (after PR interval)

» c wave - often not visible

- Closure of the tricuspid valve for CVP, mitral valve for PAOP

» v wave - atrial diastole when tricuspid or mitral valve are closed

- Produced after ventricular depolarization; QSR complex

» Read the mean of the "a" & "c" wave or

- Z-point method: read at the end of QRS complex

- Z-point is the method used when patients are in Afib or junctional rhythms

» Remember! Mechanical events (contraction) follow electrical events (depolarization)

- Lightening happens before the thunder!

Know this:

» Enlarged "a" waves = increased pressure in the atrium

- Large "a" waves in the CVP = tricuspid stenosis or high pressure in the right atrium
- Large "a" waves in the PAOP = mitral stenosis or high pressure in the left atrium
- Canon "a" waves = decreased ventricular compliance

» Enlarged "v" waves = valvular regurgitation into the atrium

- Large "v" waves in the CVP = tricuspid insufficiency or regurg, ventricular septal rupture or RV fluid overload
- Large "v" waves in the PAOP = mitral insufficiency or regurg or fluid overload

Pulmonary artery pressure (PAP)

» **Normal PA pressure = 25/10 mm Hg**

- Quarter over a dime

Causes of elevated systolic (PAS):

» **Pulmonary embolism**

» **COPD**

» **ARDS**

» **Hypoxia**

» **Pulmonary HTN**

Causes of elevated diastolic (PAD):

» **Left ventricular failure**

» **Mitral valve dysfunction**

» **Cardiac tamponade**

PA diastolic (PAD) is reflective of LVEDP except with:

» Mitral valve dysfunction

» Pulmonary HTN

» Right BBB

» Aortic insufficiency

» Pulmonic insufficiency

» Decreased LV compliance

PAOP "Wedge" pressure

» Normal 8 - 12 mm Hg

» Preload indicator

» Estimates left atrial filling pressures

» PAOP should be < PAD

» Assumes pressure & volume are directly proportional

• However, that is only in a normally compliant ventricle!

» Disproportionate increase in pressure w/ an increase in volume

» Compliance is a change in pressure for a given change in volume

Some safety tips for obtaining a PAOP reading:

» Inject air into the balloon port slowly and stop when the waveform changes

» Never inject more than 1.5 ml of air

» Stop inflating the balloon if resistance is met

» Inflate < 15 seconds

» Allow air to passively exit

» If PA waveform does not change, this may a sign of:

• Balloon rupture

• Tip of PA is in the RV or in PA

» Risk of obtaining a PAOP:

• Rupture of the pulmonary artery

• Bleeding if patients are anticoagulated

General PAOP guidelines

The PAOP will be elevated in:

» Mitral stenosis

» Mitral insufficiency

» Left ventricular failure

» Fluid/volume overload

» Cardiac tamponade

» Constrictive pericarditis

» High levels of PEEP

Lung zones

» PA Catheter placement is verified by both chest radiograph & waveforms

» PA Cath tip must be placed in Zone 3

» Signs in Zone 1 or 2:

- Damped paop waveform
- PAOP > PAD
- Absence of a and v waves

Cardiogenic Shock: LV vs. RV failure

Left Ventricular Failure	Right Ventricular Failure
Decreased CO Increased SVR Increased PAOP Decreased SvO$_2$ Dysrhythmias Crackles Decreased urine output *Wet lungs	Decreased CO (right, then left from lack of forward flow) Increased PVR Increased CVP (with a NORMAL PAOP!) JVD Hepatojugular reflux sign Peripheral edema *Clear lungs

Shock Hemodynamics

Types of Shock	CO/CI	Preload: CVP	Preload: PAOP	Afterload: SVR	Treatment
Cardiogenic (left ventricular)	Decreased	Increased or normal	Increased	Increased	+ Inotropes, Afterload reduction, Pressors
Cardiogenic (right ventricular)	Decreased	Increased	Decreased or normal	Increased	Fluids, + inotropes, Pulm vasodilators
Hypovolemic /Hemorrhage	Decreased	Decreased	Decreased	Increased	Fluids or blood
Vasodilatory /Vasoplegic	Increased or normal	Decreased or normal	Decreased or normal	Decreased	Vasopressors!
Obstructive (Tamponade)	Decreased	Increased	Increased	Increased	Pericardio-centesis, OR, fluids, + inotropes!

Vasopressors & Positive Inotropes

General thoughts:

» If a patient experiences post-op hypotension:

- Treat with volume first (at least assess for volume needs)

• If there's no improvement with volume and:

▷ The systolic is low, likely need a + inotrope (Dobutamine, Milrinone)

▷ The diastolic is low, likely need a vasopressor to tighten vascular tone

Pharmacology – Catecholamine Vasopressors & Inotropes

Drug	Alpha	Beta$_1$	Beta$_2$
Vasopressors			
Phenylephrine	++++	-	-
Norepinephrine	++++	++	-
Epinephrine	++++	++++	++
Dopamine	++ < 5 mcg/kg/min	++++ < 10 mcg/kg/min	+
	+++ > 10 mcg/kg/min		
Inotrope			
Dobutamine (+ inotrope)	+	++++	++

Location of receptors:

» Alpha – Vessels

» Beta$_1$ – Heart

» Beta$_2$ – Bronchial & vascular smooth muscle

Catecholamine Vasopressors

» Used to increase blood pressure!

» How do you know it's working? The MAP target or BP increases!

Norepinephrine (Levophed)

» Effect: ↑BP, ↑SVR, ↑C.O. (mild increase)

» Mostly alpha & some Beta$_1$

Dosing:

» 0.5 – 30 mcg/min

» Half-life is about 2 minutes

» Monitor closely for extravasation

Watch out!:

» Bradycardia, dysrhythmias, HTN, renal artery vasoconstriction

Phenylephrine (Neo-Synephrine)

» Effect: ↑ BP, ↑SVR, ↑O$_2$ consumption

» Less vasoconstriction than norepinephrine

» Pure alpha receptor stimulant

» No effect on HR to produce tachycardia

Dosing:

» 0.5 - 10 mcg/kg/min
  • 10 – 180 mcg/min

» Half-life is about 2.5 to 3 hours

» Titrate to MAP

Watch out!:

» Reflex bradycardia, dysrhythmias, HTN, chest pain, ↓ GI motility

» Monitor for extravasation

» Great drug for Cardiac Surgery if the patient has pure vasodilation (hypotension + ↓ SVR)

Epinephrine (Adrenalin)

» Effect: ↑ BP, ↑HR, ↑SVR, ↑C.O.

» Also going to increase oxygen consumption (VO_2)

» Alpha, Beta$_1$, some Beta$_2$

Dosing:

» 1 - 10 mcg/min – titrate to effect
  • 0.01 - 0.2 mcg/kg/min

» Dose dependent effects

» Always try to use the lowest dose possible

» Half-life is about 1 min

Watch out!:

» HTN, myocardial ischemia, increased O_2 consumption, tachycardia, dysrhythmias, chest pain, hypokalemia

» Monitor closely for extravasation
  • Can cause tissue necrosis
  • Central line is preferred

» Hyperglycemia; insulin resistance

Dopamine (Inotropin)

» Effect: ↑HR, ↑BP, ↑SVR, ↑C.O. (dose dependent)

» Classified as a catecholamine

» Acts on the SNS

» Positive inotropic effects

» Stimulates Beta$_1$ &
some Beta$_2$, alpha

» Monitor closely for extravasation

- Can cause tissue necrosis

Dosing:

» 0.5 - 3 mcg/kg/min –
dopaminergic receptors

» 3 - 10 mcg/kg/min – beta
effects (↑HR, BP & CO)

» > 10 mcg/kg/min – alpha
effects (↑HR & BP)

» Max 20 mcg/kg/min

» Onset of action is
about 5 minutes

» Half-life is about 2 minutes

Watch out!:

» Low doses – increased
urine output

- It dose increase renal blood flow,
but it's never been associated
with improved outcomes

- Cut it out with "renal dose
Dopamine" ☺ There is
no proven benefit!

» Higher doses – *tachycardia,*
increased SVR, increased
workload of heart (d/t
vasoconstriction), renal
ischemia, atrial &
ventricular arrhythmias

- Increased myocardial
O$_2$ consumption,
myocardial ischemia

Non-Catecholamine Vasopressors

Vasopressin (Pitressin)

» Effect: ↑BP, ↑SVR

» It's NOT a catecholamine!

- Natural anti-diuretic
hormone (ADH)

» 2nd line vasopressor, use to keep
doses of other vasopressors down

» Improved renal perfusion

» OK to give in a peripheral IV

» Use in caution in patients
with unstable CAD

» Also used in Diabetes Insipidus

Dosing:

» 0.01 – 0.1 units/min

» Half-life 10 – 20 min

Watch out!:

» Bowel ischemia, mesenteric vasoconstriction

» Decreased UOP (It's ADH!)

Methylene Blue

» Used post CBG for vasodilatory, vasoplegic hypotension

• Not first line vasopressor

» May not be able to get a pulse oximetry reading!

Dosing:

» 2 mg/kg over 20 min, then 1.5 mg/kg over 1 hour

» Maximum is 2 mg/kg

Vasopressor extravasations:

Phentolamine (Regitine)

» Alpha$_1$ blocker

» Used for vasopressor or Dilantin extravasation

• Also used for treatment of hypertension

» Phentolamine mesylate 5 – 10 mg diluted in 10 – 15 ml of saline

» Inject around infiltrated site

» Prevents necrosis & sloughing of tissue

» Limits extravasation ischemia

» Also consider warm compresses to vasodilate

Positive Inotropes

» Used to improve cardiac output & contractility

» Dobutamine & Milrinone also have some vasodilatory effects; watch the BP!

Dobutamine (Dobutrex)

» Effect: ↑ C.O./SV, ↑ HR, ↓ SVR, ↓ PAOP

» Stimulates beta receptors, $Beta_1$ (some alpha)

» Treat hypovolemia before giving Dobutamine!

Dosing:

» 2 – 20 mcg/kg/min IV (up to 40 mcg/kg/min)

» Onset 1 - 2 minutes, up to 10 min.

» Plasma half-life 2 minutes, so just decrease it or shut it off if hypotensive

» Monitor for: tachycardia, hyper/hypotension, ectopy, hypokalemia

» May develop tolerance after a few days

Milrinone (Primacor)

» Effects: ↑C.O./SV, ↓PAOP & SVR, no change in HR

» Phosphodiesterase (PDE) inhibitor
  • Inhibits the degradation of cyclic AMP in cardiac & smooth muscle

• Increases calcium influx into the myocardial cells

• Systemic & pulmonary vasodilator

• Used mostly in exacerbated heart failure

Dosing:

- » Bolus 50 mcg/kg over 10 min.

- » Maintenance: 0.25 –
  0.75 mcg/kg/min
  - • Reduce dose in renal failure

- » Long half-life – about
  2.5 hours!!!!

- » Hepatic clearance

Watch out!:

- » Vasodilatory effects – watch
  for hypotension!!!

- » Ventricular irritability –
  PVCs, hypotension, angina

- » Hypokalemia
  - • Correct hypokalemia
    & hypovolemia before
    administering!

- » Avoid in patients with severe
  valve disease or acute MI

- » Thrombocytopenia,
  bronchospasm, headache

Vasodilators

Used to decrease SVR or resistance or to decrease BP

Nitroprusside (Nipride)

- » Antihypertensive of
  nitrate origin

- » Effects: ↓MAP, SVR, PAOP, CVP,
  may ↑CO (d/t ↓afterload/SVR)

- » Arterial line preferred if titrating

- » AFTERLOAD & preload
  reducer! (Know this!)
  - • Arterial & venous vasodilator

Dosing:

- » 0.1 – 8 mcg/kg/min

- » Half-life ~ 1 min

Watch out!:

» Hypotension

- Assess BP Q 1 - 2 min until BP is stabilized

» Headache, nausea, confusion

» Hypoxia (from intrapulmonary shunt)

» Increased HR (Stimulation of baroreceptors)

» Thiocyanate poisoning (esp. if given > 72 hrs.), check level

- More common with high doses for a prolonged period of time

» Methemoglobinemia (Hgb can get converted)

» Do not use in hypotension, hypovolemia, aortic stenosis

Nitroglycerin (Tridil)

» Potent peripheral vasodilator

» Dilates arterial & venous vasculature (preload & afterload reducer!)

» Increased coronary perfusion

» Used to treat: angina, HF, HTN

Dosing:

» 5 mcg/min up to 200 mcg/min

» Can titrate pretty quickly – every 5 to 10 minutes

» Half-life is 1 – 3 min

Watch out!:

» Hypotension, bradycardia, dizziness, hypovolemia, headache, reflexive tachycardia, N/V

» In some people NTG doesn't have much effect on the BP

- May develop tolerance to NTG

» Do not use in hypotension, hypovolemia, aortic stenosis, ICP issues, constrictive pericarditis

Summary of Vasopressors, Positive Inotropes & Vasodilators

Medication	HR	MAP	C.O.	SVR	PAOP
Vasopressors					
Phenylephrine	-	↑↑↑	-	↑↑↑	↑/-
Norepinephrine	↑/-	↑↑↑	↑	↑↑↑	↑/-
Dopamine	↑↑	↑↑	↑↑	↑	↓
Epinephrine	↑↑↑	↑↑↑	↑↑↑	↑↑↑	↑/-
Vasopressin	↓/-	↑↑	↓/-	↑↑↑	↑
Positive inotropes					
Dobutamine	↑↑↑	↑/↓	↑↑↑	↓/-	↓
Milrinone	↑	↑/↓	↑↑↑	↓/-	↓
Vasodilators					
Nitroglycerin	-	↓	↑/-	↓	↓↓
Nitroprusside	-	↓↓	↑↑	↓↓	↓↓
Nicardipine		↓↓		↓	
Esmolol	↓	↓	↓/-	↓	↑/-

↑ = little effect, ↑↑ = moderate, ↑↑↑ = major, (-) = not much

You Can Do It!

Chapter 3

Procedures: Coronary Artery Bypass Grafting (CABG)

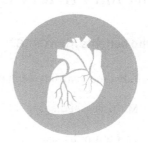

Topics covered in this chapter include:

- ► Coronary Artery Bypass Grafting (CABG) overview
- ► Cardiopulmonary Bypass (CPB)
  - • On pump/Off pump
- ► Bypass graft vessels
- ► Immediate post-operative care
- ► The Death Triad
  - • Hypothermia
  - • Acidosis
  - • Coagulopathy
- ► Other post-operative considerations
  - • Diagnostics
  - • Blood pressure control
  - • IV fluids
  - • Mechanical Ventilation
  - • Atelectasis
  - • Chest tubes
  - • Glucose control
  - • Sternal precautions

Coronary Artery Bypass Grafting (CABG) Overview

Who benefits from CABG?:

» Advanced cardiovascular disease

» Multi-vessel disease

» Left main disease

» Failed PCI

» Previous CABG with re-stenosis

» Left ventricular dysfunction

» Mechanical complications post MI
  • Ruptured papillary muscle
  • Ventricular septal wall rupture
  • Ventricular free wall rupture (poor outcomes)

Who is higher risk for CABG?:

» Females

» Over age 65

» Previous CABG

» Left ventricular dysfunction (reduced EF)

» CKD

» Diabetes

» Left main disease

» Obesity

Risk calculator for cardiac surgery (CABG or valvular):
http://riskcalc.sts.org/stswebriskcalc/

Off-Pump Cardiopulmonary Bypass (OPCPB)

Less common than on-pump bypass (CPB)

Advantages of off-pump cardiopulmonary bypass (OPCPB):

» Grafting done while heart is beating

» Decreased risk of immediate post-op stroke, atrial fibrillation, infection

» Decreased transfusions

» Decreased cost, ICU LOS, hospital LOS

» Done either minimally invasive (MIDCAB) or with median sternotomy

- ~ 15 – 20% of cases are performed minimally invasive

Who benefits from OPCPB?:

» > 70 years old

» Re-operations

» Reduced ejection fraction/ left ventricular dysfunction

Cardiopulmonary Bypass (CPB)

» Heart is arrested with circulatory support provided

» Circulatory support:

- Blood drained from the venous side (via the right atrium or femoral vein) →

- Blood is oxygenated, CO_2 removed →

- Oxygenated blood sent back to arterial circulation (via the aorta)

» Temperature is tightly controlled via the CPB circuit through a heat exchanger

- Controlled hypothermia is used during surgery

- Generally body temps down to 28 - 34°C

- Decreases O_2 demand

» Aorta is clamped once placed on CPB

» Cold cardioplegia solution (often with added bicarb) is used to arrest the heart during the surgery

- Solution is usually 4 – 8°C

- Depolarizes the cell membrane with potassium or magnesium

- Potassium-based solution protects the myocardium from cellular death

- Works by reducing myocardial metabolism in combination with hypothermia

- Raises the cardiac cellular membrane resting action potential (normal is -90 mV)

» Intra-operative anti-coagulation is required

- Heparin is most commonly used

- Monitor ACT intra-op

- Reverse with Protamine

- If the patient has HIT, can use Bivalirudin or Argatroban

Bypass Graft Vessels

» To perform a bypass, the patient needs > 1 mm vessel diameter below the stenosis with viable myocardium in the region

Bypass vessel(s) can be harvested from:

» Internal mammary artery (IMA) - aka intrathoracic arteries

- Better long term patency & survival

- *Left IMA bypass usually grafted to the LAD

- *Right IMA bypass usually grafted to the RCA
  ▷ If both IMAs used for grafting, higher potential for complicated sternal wound healing, but overall good outcomes!

» Radial artery

- Usually harvest from the non-dominant hand

- Allen test should always be performed pre-operative to assess for adequate perfusion by the ulnar artery

- Post-operative – monitor for hand ischemia

- Monitor 6 P's of radial graft-harvested hand: pain, pallor, pulse, polar (temperature), paresis & paresthesia

- *Monitor for vessel spasm
  ▷ *Often placed on Nitroglycerin or Diltiazem infusions
  ▷ Transitioned to oral by discharge

- Compressive wrap dressing is often used for 24 hours post-operative

- Monitor for bleeding, swelling & compartment syndrome (rare)

- Better outcomes compared to saphenous vein

» Saphenous vein (Leg)

- Harvesting usually done endoscopic

- Less pain and long term scarring with endoscopic

- Vein used in reverse direction because of valves in the vessel

Pertinent information to obtain from the OR regarding the surgery:

» On or off bypass?

» Cardiopulmonary bypass time?

- Longer pump time = increased risk of bleeding

- Aortic cross-clamp time

» Hemodynamic stability?

- Need for vasopressors, inotropes or vasodilators?

» Estimated blood loss (EBL)?

» Amount of IV fluids & blood products administered?

- Dryer is easier to get off the ventilator, less complications

- What products are available for the patient?

» Which vessel(s) were bypassed?

» Invasive lines & pacing wires inserted?

- Rhythm issues or complications?

- Atrial, ventricular pacing wires or both?

» Recent labs?

- Electrolytes, ABGs, coags, H & H

» Chest tubes & output?

Immediate Post-Operative Care

Immediate post-op priorities:

Hemodynamic stability

- Assess hemodynamics, lines, review infusions & doses, peripheral pulses, physical assessment, neuro assessment

Fluid balance

- Post CPB, there is considerable sympathetic nervous system (SNS) & RAAS activation

- Catecholamine release can cause tachycardia, increased BP & SVR

  ▷ Patient may have a bigger SNS response if they weren't on beta blockers pre-op

- RAAS activation causes sodium & H_2O conservation = weight gain!

  ▷ For every 1 hour on CPB, ~ 800 cc fluid gain (Third spaced)

Vasodilation (vasoplegic shock)

- Inflammation & capillary leak from CPB

- Similar to a SIRS response

- Increased inflammatory cytokines
- Decreased BP, SVR & preload
- Can last for hours post-operative

» Normothermia

- Cold = increased risk of bleeding (see additional notes in next section on hypothermia)

Recovery from anesthesia

» Full neuro assessment as the patient wakes up

Monitor for complications (dysrhythmias, electrolyte imbalance)

- Potassium & magnesium are often deficient
- Monitor for ↓ calcium especially if PRBCs given

» Bleeding & thrombocytopenia

- Thrombocytopenia caused from platelets coming in surface contact with a foreign substance (i.e. CPB machine)
- Platelet dysfunction & hemolysis of RBCs from CPB
- Hemodilution of RBCs

» Vasospasm of radial graft (if used) leading to ischemia

- 12 Lead ECG
- Monitor ST segment for ischemia, set alarms
- Diltiazem or Nitroglycerin infusions

» Monitor for vascular injury at the cannulation sites

- Monitor for hematomas, bleeding
- Monitor distal pulses

Pain management

» Usually opioids initially, then multi-modal (adding non-opioids)

Chest tubes patent & to suction

- Amount of drainage
- Assess for air leak

» Assess for early extubation (now called "liberation")

- Assess when anesthesia wears off
- Less fluid positive = easier extubation

The "Death Triad"

Emergent Immediate Post-Operative Complications:

*See Chapter 4 for a complete review of post-operative complications

» Hypothermia

- Temperature < 36° C associated with worse outcomes, increased risk of bleeding

- Normothermia is the goal
  ▷ Low temperature = decreased contractility
  ▷ Left shift on oxyhemoglobin dissociation curve

- Active re-warming if symptomatic, otherwise passive rewarm
  ▷ If re-warming is done too quickly, can see hypotension from vasodilation

- Monitor for shivering!
  ▷ Increases oxygen consumption (VO_2) by 60 – 100%!
  ▷ Meperidine 25 mg IV commonly used to control shivering

» Coagulopathy

- Assess coags (PT/INR, PTT, fibrinogen, platelets)
  ▷ Some facilities follow TEG or ROTEM (not on CSC exam)

- Bleeding, longer pump time & HTN = increased risk of bleeding

- Patients are given heparin on CPB (d/t thrombogenic nature of the circuit itself), then protamine to reverse it

- Can't always completely reverse heparin, so monitor for bleeding

- Also, watch for Heparin rebound! (See Chapter 7 – Bleeding & Coagulopathies)

- If bleeding, get the HOB to at least 30 degrees consider & increasing PEEP (decreases preload)

- Monitor chest tubes closely; clotted tubes = tamponade!

» Acidosis

- Metabolic acidosis is common

- Careful using 0.9 saline as resuscitation fluid; can exacerbate acidosis because of the chloride & lead to AKI

All components of the "Death Triad" can lead to increased risk of bleeding & higher mortality risk!

Immediate Post-operative Diagnostics

Chest Radiograph

» Verify endotracheal
tube placement

- Tip of tube should sit 3 - 4 cm
  ± 2 cm above the carina

» Verify line placement

- Central line, gastric tubes

» Identify pneumo or hemothorax

» Verify IABP catheter placement

- Tip should sit at the 2nd to
  3rd intercostal space

- Below the subclavian, but
  above the renal arteries

12 Lead ECG

» Monitor ST segment for
ischemic changes

» New Q waves are a bad sign

» Bedside ST segment monitoring
– good, but get false alarms

Labs - as indicated:

» ABG

» SvO_2/$ScvO_2$

- Assesses how the patient
  is utilizing oxygen

- Normal 65 – 75% (see the
  hemodynamics chapter
  for more info)

» Chemistry – closely watch
potassium, magnesium, calcium

» Coags, hemoglobin, platelets,
fibrinogen – if bleeding

» Follow lactate levels if concerns
for hypoperfusion or shock

Other Post-operative Monitoring Considerations

Blood Pressure control

» General MAP target 60 – 80 mm Hg, maybe up to 90 mm Hg

- Establish specific patient target with CT surgeon or provider

- Higher for chronic HTN or renal issues

- Lower for systolic heart failure with reduced EF, mitral valve replacement, bleeding

» ↑ BP = increased risk of bleeding

» Control with pain meds or sedation, vasodilators

» If hypotensive, consider reasons why:

- Bleeding

- Hypovolemia

- Vasodilated from inflammation

- Re-warming induced vasodilation

- Low cardiac output

IV fluid management

» If hypotensive & not bleeding post-op, it's common to give fluids

» Reminder, tons of third spacing & capillary leak post-op!!!

» Crystalloids, colloids or blood

- Lactated ringers or Plasmalyte-A are becoming the "go to" fluid choices

- Normosol can also be considered
  ▷ Contains potassium & magnesium, less chloride than 0.9 saline

Mechanical Ventilation

» SpO$_2$ & EtCO$_2$ are great surrogates to oxygen/ventilation

- Normal EtCO$_2$ = 35 – 45 mm Hg (assuming normal V/Q matching)

Vent settings:

» Mode: volume or pressure (volume is more commonly used)

» Tidal volume: Dosed on predicted body weight!

- 6 - 8 ml/kg PBW

- If concern for lung injury, use less tidal volume (more toward 6 ml/kg)

» Set rate: Usually 10 – 14 bpm

» PEEP: Start with +5 cm H_2O

» Goal is early extubation
   within 4 – 8 hours post-op

» Challenges: patient's age,
   anesthesia used, level of sedation

» Benefits of early extubation?

- ↓ hospital LOS

- ↓ pulmonary complications

- Early mobility

To successfully liberate from the ventilator:

» Awake! Sedation
   & neuromuscular
   blockade worn off

» Able to lift head off the bed

» Pain needs to be controlled

» Hemodynamically stable

» Temperature close to
   normothermia

» Pass SBT – monitor
   ABG or SpO_2/$EtCO_2$

- SBT usually done on CPAP
   or pressure support

- Can assess negative
   inspiratory force (NIF)

- Assess minute ventilation

Post-extubation:

» Monitor $EtCO_2$ & SpO_2

- Rising $EtCO_2$ =
   hypoventilation/tired

- Decreasing $EtCO_2$ =
   hyperventilation

- Pain control

- Ambulate!!!!

- If the patient decompensates,
   consider:
   ▷ High flow nasal cannula
      (oxygenation issue)
   ▷ BiPAP (ventilation issue)
      - With BiPAP, watch for
         aspiration

Not ready to extubate:

- Gets hemodynamically
   unstable during SBT

- VS changes: tachycardia, ↑RR
   with increased work of breathing

- Gets acidotic (↓pH, ↑CO_2)

- Desaturations

- Increasing $EtCO_2$

Atelectasis*

» It's a major issue!

» At risk: smokers, COPD, pain issues (hypoventilation), immobility

» May hear ↓ breath sounds, crackles, wheezing

» Can get mucus plugs

» May have tachycardia with a low grade temp

» Pulmonary toilet, cough & deep breath

- Incentive spirometer every hour while awake

» Manage pain; chest/ sternal splinting

» Ambulate!

Pain

» Multi-modal approach preferred

» Non-opioid as a foundation (often scheduled vs. prn)

» Opioids for moderate to severe pain; fentanyl commonly used while intubated

» May see nausea with pain, use an anti-emetic

Chest tubes

» Mediastinal tubes placed to – 20 cm H_2O or dry suction

» 2 – 3 tubes are typical

- Pleural tubes are only placed if the pleural space was opened in the OR

» Usually removed within 24 – 72 hours post-operative

» Tidaling is normal

- Fluctuation with breathing in the water seal/air leak chamber

» Purpose is to assist with clearance of blood from the pericardial space

- Prevents cardiac tamponade

- Important to maintain patency of the chest tubes!

- Do not strip tubes – creates a lot of negative pressure within the thoracic cavity!

- Avoid dependent loops!

Spontaneously breathing patient:

» Water level rises during inspiration, falls during exhalation

» Opposite for mechanically ventilated patient

- If tidaling is not present: assess for obstructing in the tubing (clot or kink)

Signs of a pneumothorax:

» Bubbles in the water seal/ air leak chamber

» First assess for a loose connection or break in the system

- Check connections (assessing for a system air leak) – if that doesn't resolve bubbling, it may be a patient air leak

- Chest radiograph will verify if there is a pneumothorax (patient air leak)

» Discontinue chest tubes when drainage is ~ < 100 ml for 4 hours

- Pre-medicate for pain prior to removal

- When discontinuing the chest tube(s), elevate HOB 20 – 30 degrees, instruct the patient to deep breathe & exhale, gently discontinue the tube

- Obtain a chest radiograph post removal

Dysrhythmias/blocks

» Careful monitoring of electrolytes

- Potassium & magnesium

- More prone to arrhythmias if either are low

» With aortic or mitral valve replacement, monitor for heart block!

- Be prepared to pace if heart block develops!

» Atrial fibrillation is covered in Chapter 8 – Electrical Issues

Glucose control; goal 140 – 180 mg/dL

» Hyperglycemia is common post CPB

  • Catecholamine & stress response

» Hyperglycemia is associated with poor outcomes

» Better control reduces wound infections & promotes healing

» Use an insulin infusion protocol for the first 12 – 24 hours, then transition to SQ insulin as needed

» Always know what the patient's potassium is before giving insulin!

  • Insulin transports potassium into the cell

» If Epinephrine infusion is used for hemodynamic support, monitor for hyperglycemia!

  • Remember Epi is an exogenous catecholamine, so it will increase glucose levels!

» Hypoglycemia can be deadly!!!!

  • Although it's not common post CPB, avoid it!!!

Sternal precautions

» The sternum is reinforced with special sternal wires

» Required to prevent dehiscence of the sternum

» If not followed can lead to sternal wound infections

» Instruct the patient NOT to:

  • Lift more than 5 - 8 pounds

  • Push or pull with their arms

  • Reach behind their back, both arms out to the side or overhead

Other considerations:

» Mobilize as early as possible!

» Discontinue central lines when hemodynamically stable & off vasopressors, inotropes & vasodilators

» Discontinue bladder catheter asap

» Incisions are usually covered with a sterile dressing for 24 hours

- After 24 hours, remove dressing & keep incisions open to air if there's no drainage

- Ace wraps are often used with radial artery & saphenous vein graft sites; remove after 24 – 48 hours

» VTE prophylaxis with SCDs

- Can also use UFH or LMWH for high risk patients

» GI prophylaxis for high risk patients only!

You Can Do It!

Chapter 4

Cardiovascular Complications of Cardiac Surgery

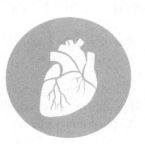

Topics covered in this section include:

- ► Cardiogenic shock
- ► Myocardial stunning
- ► Post-Myocardial infarction
- ► Intra-Aortic Balloon Pump (IABP)
- ► Short-term ventricular assist devices (VADs)
- ► Vasoplegic (vasodilatory) Shock
- ► Right heart failure
- ► Post-operative dysrhythmias
- ► Cardiac Tamponade
- ► Open chest from the OR
- ► Pericarditis
- ► Malignant Hyperthermia
- ► Cardiac Arrest

Cardiogenic Shock

» The mortality of shock is about 40 – 50 %

» Classic clinical picture – hypotension/tachycardia, +/- pulmonary edema

» Post-cardiac surgery with CPB, the CO may decline for the 1st 4 – 6 hours

» A pulmonary artery catheter can be helpful in guiding therapy (although the data are mixed)

» Consider ECHO to evaluate wall motion, EF & other potential causes of cardiogenic shock post-operatively

Causes of left ventricular dysfunction post CABG:

» Decreased preload

- Hypovolemia
- Blood loss
- Vasodilation

» Peri-operative/post-op MI

» Arrhythmias

- Tachycardia
- Loss of A-V synchrony, atrial kick

- Atrial fibrillation
  ▷ NOT tolerated if the patient has pre-operative ↓ EF or left ventricular hypertrophy (LVH)

» Cardioplegia injury

» Myocardial stunning

» Increased afterload

- Hypertension (vasoconstriction)

» Cardiac Tamponade

Key diagnostics to determine cause:

» Pulmonary Artery Catheter/ Hemodynamic Measurements

» Echocardiogram

- TEE/TTE, may see:
  ▷ Hypokinetic or akinetic wall motion

▷ Reduced ejection fraction
▷ Acute valvular regurgitation

» 12 Lead ECG

- Assess for new Q waves
- ST segment changes

Clinical signs:

» Tachycardia

» Hypotension

» S3 heart sound

» Pulmonary edema

» Dysrhythmias

» Signs of decreased perfusion

» Decreased UOP

- oliguria < 0.5 ml/kg/hr

» Metabolic acidosis

» Elevated lactate

Hemodynamics: (KNOW this!!!!)

» Tachycardia

- May not see if the patient received beta blockers

» Hypotension (MAP < 60 mm Hg)

» Low C.O. & C.I. (< 2.2 L/min/m^2)

» Elevated SVR, often > 1400 dynes/sec/cm^{-5}

» Elevated RAP/CVP

» Elevated PAOP (> 12 mm Hg)

» Decreased SvO$_2$ (< 65%)

Other diagnostics:

» Troponin-I

- It will be elevated after cardiac surgery, so its usefulness is limited

» Cardiac Catheterization

- If graft occlusion is suspected

- Percutaneous Coronary Intervention (PCI) for reperfusion

- Grafts can be stented

» ABG

- Mixed respiratory & metabolic acidosis; hypoxemia

- Lactic acidosis due to decreased perfusion & anaerobic metabolism

» Lactate levels

- Normal is < 2 mmol/L; > 4 – 5 mmol/L is associated with poor outcomes

- Elevated in states of hypoperfusion

- May also see an elevation if receiving an Epinephrine infusion!

» Chest x-ray

- Pulmonary congestion

- May note opacity due to enlarged pulmonary vasculature

» BUN/Creatinine

- Monitor urine output closely

- High risk for acute kidney injury

- Remember creatinine is a late indicator!
  ▷ BUN is non-specific

» Monitor other organs for dysfunction & failure

Treatment:

» Optimize preload, but don't over-resuscitate with fluid!

» Optimize HR with pacing if appropriate

- Usually like HR ~ 80 or so

» + Inotrope to improve contractility

- i.e. Dobutamine, Milrinone, Epi, Norepi

- Use Milrinone cautiously in patients with renal dysfunction

» Afterload reduction / venous vasodilators (i.e. NTG)

» Vasopressors to support blood pressure

- Use with caution as they will increase the SVR & increase the workload of the heart

» If fluid overloaded, consider diuretics (as perfusion allows)

» **Mechanical support (i.e. IABP, Impella)**

- I want to list this option first!!!!

- IABP info can be found in next few pages

Cardiogenic Pulmonary Edema

» Fluid in the alveolus d/t increased alveolar hydrostatic pressures

» Impaired gas exchange, hypercapnia

» Hypoxemia, S3 heart sound, shortness of breath, anxiety, crackles, pink frothy sputum, may have a murmur

Causes:

» Transfusion overload (TACO), peri/post-op myocardial infarction, heart failure, hypertension, mitral regurgitation, tamponade

Treatment:

» Loop diuretics (preload reducer)

» Morphine (preload & afterload reducer)

» Vasodilator

» Consider + Inotrope (i.e. Dobutamine) to improve contractility

» Oxygen support, may need mechanical ventilation

» Can use Bi-PAP for non-invasive ventilation support

  • Will also decrease preload

» Ultrafiltration if non-responsive

Myocardial Stunning / Low Cardiac Output Syndrome

» Reversible low cardiac output state after CPB

  • Usually lasts 4 – 6 hours post CPB, sometimes longer

  • Impaired myocardial function after temporary ischemia

  • Contractility impaired after cross-clamping of the aorta during surgery

» What contributes to it?

  • Low EF pre-op

  • Long CPB time

  • Reperfusion injury post CPB

  • Acidosis

  • Myocardial edema

» Monitor for signs similar to cardiogenic shock:

  • Decreased CO/CI

  • Increasing SVR (vasoconstriction to compensate)

  • Increasing filling pressures (PAOP/CVP)

  • Decreasing SvO_2

» May need + inotrope

  • Dobutamine or Milrinone

  • May consider Epinephrine

» Consider cardiac assist device to temporarily support the LV

  • IABP or Impella

Post-Operative Myocardial Infarction

» Grafts can acutely close, thrombose/clot, or develop vasospasm leading to myocardial ischemia &/or infarction

» Over-sewing of graft, surgical injuries

» Can be caused from a coronary air embolism from CPB

» Over time, grafts can develop atherosclerotic plaque causing stenosis & occlusion (obviously, not immediate post-op)

» Who is at risk?

- Re-Operation, Pre-Op MI, failed PCI, left main, ↓EF pre-op

» Challenging to make diagnosis based on 12 Lead ECG & troponin

» 12 Lead ECG:

- May have ST changes due inflammation of the pericardium

- New left BBB is ominous

- Assess for reciprocal changes

- Monitor for Q waves post-op
  ▷ Associated with poor outcome
  ▷ Can be a sign of poor distal perfusion after grafting

» Cardiac Enzymes/Biomarkers:

- Cardiac enzymes will be elevated from the procedure

- Troponin-I or CK-MB that is 5 x normal may be indicative of post-op MI

» Treatment:

- Get an ECHO to assess wall motion

- Start anti-platelet therapy (aspirin or Clopidogrel)

- Start beta blocker & nitroglycerin

Revascularize!!!

- Consider PCI

- Also may consider re-operation if a large area of the myocardium is at risk

- IABP if the patient is hemodynamically unstable

- If vasospasm is suspected, administer Nitroglycerin or Diltiazem IV or PO

- Discharge: Will go home on anti-platelet therapy & statins

Intra-Aortic Balloon Counterpulsation IABC/IABP

» Used in cardiogenic shock

- Pre-CABG for high risk patients

- Difficulty weaning from CPB

- Post CABG & decompensated heart failure

» Balloon <u>inflates</u> at the onset of <u>diastole</u>

- Inflates at the dicrotic notch

- Dicrotic notch signifies closure of the aortic valve

- Coronary arteries are perfused during diastole

- Increases perfusion

» Balloon <u>deflates</u> right before <u>systole</u>

- Benefit: There's less resistance to pump against

- Afterload or resistance to ejection is reduced

Theoretical benefits of IABP:

» Increased coronary artery perfusion

» Increased perfusion to organs

» Increased myocardial O_2 supply

» Increased myocardial O_2 supply

» Decreased myocardial O_2 demand

» Decreased afterload

If the Augmentation pressure is low:

» Check catheter position

» Assess timing

» Correct hypovolemia

Position of IABP catheter:

» Positioned between the 2nd & 3rd intercostal space

- Below the left subclavian artery

- Above the renal arteries

- Verified by chest radiograph

» Palpate left radial pulse

- If unable to palpate, catheter is positioned too high

» Monitor urine output closely

- If dropping, catheter may be positioned too low

» Femoral artery insertion is common

- Can also insert brachial or transthoracic
- Monitor pulses distal to the insertion site!!!!

Contraindications for IABP:

» Aortic insufficiency

» Aortic aneurysm

» Aortic calcifications (can cause balloon rupture)

Complications of IABP:

» Limb ischemia

- Monitor distal pulses closely

» Incorrect timing

» Malposition

» Renal artery occlusion (if positioned too low)

» Infection

» Balloon rupture

- Assess the helium tubing; it should be clear

- If you see red flecks or blood, there is a rupture in the balloon
- Place in standby mode, notify the provider & prepare to discontinue within 30 min
- Assess hemodynamics for need of balloon catheter replacement

» Bleeding

- At the insertion site
- Thrombocytopenia; platelet damage from the pulsation of the device

Mechanical Circulatory Devices

Short-term/Temporary ventricular assist devices (VADs)

» Percutaneous or surgically implanted

» Continuous flow to offload the ventricle(s)

» Left ventricular assist devices (LVADs) are the most common

- Must have adequate right ventricular function

- Can also use a right ventricular assist device (RVAD)
  ▷ Used when medical therapy has been maximized & failed

- Biventricular assist device (BiVAD)

» Can be used as:

- Bridge to recovery
  ▷ Acute support, unable to wean off cardiopulmonary bypass
  ▷ Reversible LV dysfunction from MI or cardiogenic shock
  ▷ Explanted post-operative

- Bridge to transplant
  ▷ Used longer term until the patient receives a heart transplant
  ▷ Basically, they can't live without the VAD

Surgically implanted VADs

Example: HeartMate 3™

» General concept of LVAD

- Blood → LV → inflow cannula → pump → outflow cannula → aorta

- The pump is usually implanted above the diaphragm

- Unloads the workload of the left ventricle

» Anticoagulation needed

Post-Operative VAD placement considerations

» Immediate concerns:

» Bleeding!

- Assess coags for coagulopathy

» Stroke

» RV failure – monitor closely for this!

- It is imperative to have adequate right to left ventricular forward flow!

- CVP/RAP will rise if the RV is failing

- May need volume to maximize preload

- Also consider + inotrope (Milrinone or Dobutamine)
  ▷ Caution with hypotension with Milrinone

- Pulmonary vasodilators can also be helpful (Inhaled Epoprostenol (Flolan) or Nitric Oxide (iNO = $$))

» Arrhythmias

Longer term VAD concerns:

» Thrombosis (will need anticoagulation)

- VTE prophylaxis

» Bleeding

» Infection

» Late RV dysfunction

Percutaneous VADs

Examples:

» Impella

- Axial pump

- Inserted through a catheter

- Catheter goes from femoral artery → cross aortic valve → left ventricle

- Blood is propelled from the LV to the aorta, offloading the workload of the LV

- 2 sizes: 2.5 (flow rate up to 2.5 L/min) or 5.0 (flow rate up to 5 L/min)

- Also have Impella RP (right ventricular support); flow rate ~ 4 L/min

» TandemHeart

- Left atrium-to-femoral artery bypass

- 2 cannulas

- Femoral vein → IVC → right atrium, trans-septal puncture → left atrium

- Oxygenated blood from the left atrium → impeller → femoral artery via arterial cannula

- Flow assistance up to 4 L/min

» Anticoagulation required

- Once surgical bleeding is under control

Extracorporeal Membrane Oxygenation (ECMO)

» Technically, it's a form of Cardiopulmonary Bypass

» Newer devices are easy, small & portable

» Modes of ECMO:

- Veno-Venous ECMO (V-V ECMO)
  ▷ Used for Pulmonary failure (i.e. ARDS, influenza)
  ▷ Blood is oxygenated, CO_2 can be removed
  ▷ Short term support
  ▷ Although some patients will require support for days to weeks (let's be honest, months in some people)

- Venous-Arterial ECMO (V-A ECMO)
  - ▷ Heart & lungs are bypassed
  - ▷ Used for Cardiac or Cardiopulmonary failure
- ▷ Short term support
- ▷ Blood from central vein → gas exchanger (oxygenates & removes CO_2) → pump → arterial circulation

Vasoplegic Shock

» A.k.a. vasodilatory or distributive shock

» Low SVR with normal or high cardiac output

» Thought to be caused from:

- SIRS from ischemia
- Reperfusion injury
- Increased nitric oxide (NO) release causing vasodilation

- Endotoxins
- Contact with the CPB circuit
- May also see this post VAD placement

» At risk:

- Pre-operative ↓EF
- Pre-op ACE-inhibitor use
- Long aortic cross clamp time

Treatment:

» On the exam, look for a scenario with normal CO, low SVR & BP, normal filling pressures... choose the vasopressor!!!!!

» Start a low-dose vasopressor!

- Norepinephrine infusion
  - ▷ Has both alpha & beta$_1$ properties
- Add Vasopressin infusion if needed
  - ▷ Due to arginine-vasopressin deficiency

- Methylene Blue
  - ▷ If thought to be due to increased nitric oxide production
  - ▷ Not a 1st line treatment
  - ▷ Cardiac Surgeons might try Methylene Blue if the patient is not responding to vasopressors
  - ▷ 1.5 mg/kg IV over an hour

» Ensure adequate volume resuscitation, but don't over-resuscitate!

- Monitor for pulmonary issues with fluid

Right Ventricular Failure

» In the setting of RV failure, the RV dilates with damage

» Right ventricular fluid overload causes acute tricuspid regurgitation

Symptoms:

» Tachycardia

» Hypotension

» + JVD (with clear lungs)

» **Rising CVP/RAP, normal PAOP**
  - Will see large "v" waves on the CVP tracing

» May see pulmonary hypertension, but not always

» ↑ PVR

» Tricuspid regurgitation

» **Physiology:** ↑CVP → Tricuspid regurg → ↓RV stroke volume, ↓RV CO → ↑pressure on septal wall → LV compression! → ↓LV CO

Causes:

» Ischemia/Reperfusion Syndrome post-op

» Prolonged CPB

» Increased PVR after coming off CPB

» Poor myocardial protection intra-op

» Pre-existing RV dysfunction

» Graft failure

» Air embolism

» Pulmonary embolism

» Pre-existing pulmonary hypertension

Diagnostics:

» Consider Echocardiogram

» Right heart pressures from PA cath:
  - ↑ CVP/RAP
  - ↑ PA pressures (may not always be elevated)
  - ↑ PVR

Treatment:

» Optimize preload!

- Caution with fluid as it can lead to lung injury

- Target a higher CVP goal – be sure to establish the goal with the team!
  ▷ In some cases the CVP goal is > 15 mm Hg

» + Inotrope (increase contractility) – i.e. Dobutamine, Milrinone

» If continued hypotension, start a vasopressor like norepinephrine

» Minimize PEEP on the ventilator

» Inhaled pulmonary vasodilators

- Epoprostenol nebulized
  ▷ Very short half-life!

- Nitric oxide
  ▷ Gas administered via ventilator circuit
  ▷ Up to 40 PPM

» IABP if needed

» In severe cases (last resource) a right ventricular assist device (RVAD) can be used

Avoid medications that lower preload:

» Nitrates, morphine, beta blockers, diuretics

» RV is stunned & becomes **preload dependent!**

» Minimize the use of PEEP, may impede venous return

» Avoid hypoxia, acidosis or ↑CO_2

Post-Operative Dysrhythmias

» Post-operative atrial fibrillation is the most common

» See Chapter 8 on Electrical Issues for atrial fibrillation coverage

» Get a 12 Lead ECG

» Consider an atrial ECG if it's difficult to distinguish the rhythm

» Rule out cardiac or pulmonary causes of the arrhythmia

Other thoughts:

» Check & replace electrolytes!!!

» Hypokalemia – if the K^+ < 3.5, there is a greater risk of dysrhythmias!

» Hypomagnesemia is also common

» Ventricular dysrhythmias

• PVCs, non-sustained ventricular tachycardia can be caused from reperfusion

• Assess magnesium!

Cardiac Tamponade

» The pericardial space normally contains 20 – 50 ml of pericardial fluid

2 layers of pericardium:

» Parietal (outer)

» Visceral (inner)

Causes of tamponade:

» Bleeding post CABG

» Undrained blood or clots in the thoracic cavity

» Clotted chest tubes

» Myocardial edema

• Can see this when the surgeon closes the chest, the patient becomes HD unstable from myocardial compression from organ edema

» Pericardial effusion

• It's common post CABG

• Most are small & asymptomatic

• Some can cause tamponade!

» Pericarditis

» Myocardial rupture

» Uremia (renal failure patients)

Diagnostic imaging:

» Echocardiogram

» Chest x-ray

• Widened mediastinum

• Enlarged cardiac silhouette

• Dilated aorta, compressed atria – leads to decreased venous return

Signs of cardiac tamponade:

» Large mediastinal chest tube output, then...

» Sudden decrease in chest tube drainage

• Think: chest tubes clotted!

Beck's Triad:

» Elevated CVP w/JVD

» Hypotension from ↓CO

» Muffled heart sounds

Other symptoms:

» Shortness of breath

» Tachycardia

» Decreased cardiac output

» ↓SvO$_2$

» Narrowed pulse pressure

- Systolic pressure falls, diastolic pressure rises

» Increased filling pressures

» Pulsus paradoxus

- > 10 mm Hg drop in BP during inspiration

» Equalization of cardiac filling pressures

- CVP = PAOP (or PAD if you don't follow PAOP)

- Intracardiac pressures "Rise and Equalize"

» Electrical alternans

» Decreased urine output

» Metabolic acidosis

» Cardiac arrest

Treatment:

» Prevention

- Positioning & turning with HOB elevation (↓preload)

- Maintain patent chest tubes

» Suction chest tubes (provider)

» Administer fluid, + inotrope, vasopressor

» Minimize PEEP

» Pericardiocentesis

- Risk: Laceration of coronary artery

» Re-sternotomy – emergency at the bedside or the OR

- More common than pericardiocentesis

- Keep the field sterile!!!!

- Done for bleeding, tamponade or cardiac arrest (if Vfib unresponsive to defib)

Goals:

- Relieve pressure
- Maximize cardiac filling

- Locate & control source of bleeding
- Assess for coagulopathy

Open Chest from the OR

» Delayed sternal closure; avoid any myocardial compression

- Impairment of venous return leading to ↓CO

» Reasons the chest may be left open post-operative:

- Low cardiac output
- Intractable bleeding
- Myocardial edema
- Arrhythmia
- Cardiac tamponade
- VAD placement

» Who is at risk?:

- Elderly
- Combined surgeries (CABG + valve)
- Coagulopathy
- Long CPB or aortic cross clamp times

- Pre-operative anti-platelet meds
- Pre-operative MI

» Sterile, occlusive dressing left over the open chest

- Ioban® over the chest, pack with Esmark
- Do NOT put defib pads on top of the Ioban® dressing, energy can arc

» Leave patient in the supine position with minimal turning

» Treatment: aggressive diuresis to reduce the edema

- Usually close within 2 – 5 days

» If the patient has an arrest, access the chest, internal massage & defibrillate

» Higher risk for sternal wound infections

Pericarditis

» Post-pericardiotomy syndrome

» Chest pain is the #1 complaint

» Can develop days to weeks after surgery

» Inflammation of the pericardial sac

Symptoms:

» Fever

» Pleuritic pain worse with cough, inspiration; relieved by leaning forward

» Non-specific ST segment changes in the precordial leads

» Diffuse ST segment elevation on 12 lead ECG

Treatment:

» Supportive

» Anti-inflammatory meds
  • Ibuprofen, colchicine, aspirin
  • Monitor renal function closely!!!

» Steroids

» If bacterial, antibiotics

Malignant Hyperthermia

» Severe reaction & hypermetabolic state in response to anesthesia
  • Often genetic pre-disposition
  • Ca^{++} is released from muscles

» Observe significant hyperthermia, tachycardia, rigors, muscle spasms
  • Can also see rhabdomyolysis, hyperkalemia & metabolic acidosis

» Very challenging to recognize in the OR due to CPB & cooling

Treatment:

» Dantrolene 2.5 mg/kg IV

» Blocks Ca^{++} release

» Regulate the patient's temperature
  • Surface cooling or catheters
  • Avoid rapid rewarming

Cardiac Arrest & Resuscitation

» *For the CSC exam, they added CALS for resuscitation

» Cardiac arrest is actually rare post cardiac surgery

» Survival is higher in the Cardiac Surgery population compared to other hospitalized patients

CALS: Cardiac Surgery Advanced Life Support

Figure out cause asap!

» If **tamponade** or **bleeding:**

- Plan for resternotomy

- Open chest massage provides better cardiac output

» If **Vfib:**

- 3 stacked shocks

- Plan for resternotomy; external chest compressions for support alternating every 2 minutes with defibrillation

- Caution with Epinephrine (adrenaline) – do not give unless a senior provider advises to do so

General ACLS, big picture:

» Early CPR with **minimal** interruptions

» Compressions of good quality

- 100 - 120/minute

- 2 - 2.4 inch depth

» Early defibrillation

» Avoid hyperventilation – ventilate 10 breaths/min

- ↑ ventilation leads to ↑ intrathoracic pressure, leads to ↓ venous return, leads to ineffective CPR

» Figure out cause

» Causes to consider in the cardiac surgery patient:

- Hypothermia

- Electrolyte imbalances

- Acidosis

- Myocardial ischemia

- Hypoxia

- R on T, Torsades

- Tamponade

- Bleeding

- Pulmonary embolism

- Air embolism (rare, would likely see this in the OR)

Ventricular Fibrillation

» <u>S</u>hock (if readily available); Repeat Q 2 min.

» <u>C</u>PR for 2 min

» <u>R</u>hythm check - shock if warranted

» <u>E</u>pi 1mg IV Q 3-5 min*

» <u>A</u>miodarone 300 mg IV; repeat bolus 150 mg IV if still in VF/VT

» <u>M</u>edications (other):   Lidocaine 1.0 - 1.5 mg/kg IV

Caution with Epinephrine in the setting of post-operative Cardiopulmonary bypass grafting!!!!

Torsades de Pointes

» Shift in axis

» Caused by hypomagnesemia, prolonged QT (> 480 msec), multiple medications, inappropriate pacing (sensing)

» Treatment: Magnesium Sulfate 1 - 2 grams IV (diluted)

» Magnesium antagonist: Calcium Chloride

» Always consider meds that may prolong the QT!

PEA (pulseless electrical activity)/Asystole

» <u>P</u>ump: Start compressions

» <u>E</u>pinephrine 1mg IV Q 3 - 5 min (cautious!)

» <u>A</u>ssess causes

5 H's:

» Hypovolemia

» Hypoxia

» Hypo/Hyperkalemia

» H+ ion (acidosis)

» Hypothermia

5 T's:

» Thrombus:
  • MI
  • PE

» Tension pneumothorax

» Tamponade

» Toxicology (drug OD)

Note: See Chapter 8 for information on pacing!

Capnography during resuscitation

» Used as a marker of perfusion, CPR quality (with caution) & identification of ROSC

» Normal $PEtCO_2$ 35 - 45 mm Hg

- Minimum goal > 10 mm Hg during CPR

- If less than 10 mm Hg, improve quality of compressions

- If rapid increase in $PEtCO_2$, may be a sign of ROSC

- If consistently < 10 mm Hg in the setting of adequate compressions, discuss termination of resuscitation efforts
  ▷ If consistently < 10 mm Hg, consider the possibility of pulmonary embolism

Post Cardiac Arrest Care

» Optimize hemodynamics

- Avoid hypotension

- Avoid hypoxemia or hyperoxemia

» Reperfusion

- Does the patient need to go to the Cath lab?

» Targeted Temperature Management

- 32 - 36°C for 24 hours; cardiac surgery may opt for 36°C

- Recommended for all rhythms & in-hospital arrest

- Obviously, a discussion would need to happen in the cardiac surgery patient because of bleeding risk

» Cooling has never been studied in post-arrest Cardiac Surgery patients, but it may be reasonable to consider

Purpose of TTM: To minimize reperfusion injury that leads to neurologic damage

NEURO protective and minimizes:

» Depleted stores of O_2 & glucose

» Intracellular calcium influx

» Formation of O_2 free radicals

» Release of glutamate

» Intracellular acidosis

» Disruption in blood brain barrier

» Mitochondrial injury

» Apoptosis

PEARLS:

» 32° C – 36° C for 24 hours

» Only in patients remaining comatose post cardiac arrest

» AHA class I recommendation for all rhythms

» Neuro protective

» Avoid fever post TTM for at least 48 hours

» Rewarm slowly

Side effects of cooling:

» Shivering**

» Bradycardia (seen more with 32° C – 34° C range)

  • Only treat if hypotensive

» Vasoconstriction induced hypertension

» Diuresis (seen more with 32° C – 34° C range)

» Hypokalemia/ electrolyte shifting (seen more with 32° C – 34° C range)

» Elevated lactate

  • Clears when the patient rewarms

You Can Do It!

Chapter 5

Valvular Surgery & Procedures

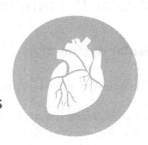

Topics covered in this chapter include:

- Valvular Dysfunction & Murmurs
- Mitral Valve Dysfunction
  - Mitral Stenosis & Regurgitation/Insufficiency
  - Transcatheter procedures: MitraClip, Valvuloplasty
  - Immediate post-operative concerns Mitral Valve Repair or Replacement
- Aortic Valve Dysfunction
  - Aortic Stenosis & Regurgitation/Insufficiency
  - Transcatheter procedures: TAVR
  - Immediate post-operative concerns Aortic Valve Replacement
- Tricuspid & Pulmonic Valve Dysfunction
- Infective Endocarditis

Valvular Dysfunction & Murmurs

Valvular dysfunction

» Is either acquired or congenital

» Can be acute (regurgitation/insufficiency) or chronic (stenosis or regurgitation)

» It is usually slow & progressive over time

» FYI – the terms "regurgitation" & "insufficiency" are often used interchangeably

Murmurs - 2 causes:

Stenosis

» Narrowed opening of the valve usually caused from atherosclerotic plaque

» Forward flow of blood through stenotic <u>open</u> valves

» Typically lower pitched murmurs

Regurgitation/Insufficiency

» Incompetent valve leaflet that doesn't completely close

» Allows for backward flow of blood

» Backward flow through incompetent <u>closed</u> valves

» Murmurs are high pitched except murmurs of stenosis

Systolic murmurs

» Pulmonic & aortic sten<u>O</u>sis are systolic murmurs...

   • Murmurs of sten<u>O</u>sis are auscultated when valves are <u>O</u>pen!

   • The pulmonic & aortic valves are <u>O</u>pen during systole

   • Therefore, they are systolic murmurs!

» Tricuspid & mitral regurg/insufficiency are systolic murmurs...

- Murmurs of insufficiency are auscultated when valves are closed!

- The tricuspid & mitral valves are closed during systole

- Therefore, they are systolic murmurs!

» Auscultate on and between S1 & S2 (during systole)

- S1 - murmur - S2

Diastolic murmurs

» Tricuspid & mitral sten<u>O</u>sis are diastolic murmurs...

- Murmurs of sten<u>O</u>sis are auscultated when valves are <u>O</u>pen!

- The tricuspid & mitral valves are <u>O</u>pen during diastole

- Therefore, they are diastolic murmurs!

» Pulmonary & aortic regurgitation/insufficiency are diastolic murmurs...

- Murmurs of insufficiency are auscultated when valves are closed!

- The pulmonic & aortic valves are closed during diastole

- Therefore, they are diastolic murmurs

» Auscultate after S2 (during diastole)

- S1 - S2 - murmur

Type of murmur	Systolic or Diastolic?	Location
Mitral Stenosis	Diastolic	5th ICS, MCL
Mitral Regurg	Systolic	5th ICS, MCL
Aortic Stenosis	Systolic	2nd ICS, RSB
Aortic Regurg	Diastolic	2nd ICS, RSB

All Valvular Dysfunction:

Valvular diagnosis

» Echocardiogram** (Gold standard)

- Transthoracic
- Transesophageal

Other diagnostics that may be helpful:

» Cardiac catheterization

- Is it ischemic in nature?
- Want to identify if the patient has:
  ▷ ↑LVEDP, ↑atrial pressure, ↑PAOP, ↓CO

» 12 lead ECG

- Assess for signs of atrial & ventricular hypertrophy

» Chest Radiograph

- Assess for atrial & ventricular enlargement
- Pulmonary venous congestion
- Enlarged heart/heart failure

» Treat heart failure if present:

- ACE inhibitor, ARB or ARNI
- Beta blocker (blunt the SNS & RAAS)
- Diuretics
- Afterload reduction

Mitral Valve Dysfunction

The Mitral Valve

» Left heart A-V valve

» Open during diastole, closed during systole

» It's a bicuspid valve with 2 leaflets

- Large anterior leaflet with a smaller posterior leaflet

» Chordae tendineae & papillary muscles assist with valve opening & closure with pressure changes

Mitral insufficiency/regurgitation (MR)

» Systolic murmur caused from an incompetent leaflet of the mitral valve

» Backward flow of blood into the left atrium

- High left atrial volume & pressure
- Can lead to left atrial enlargement

- Pulmonary congestion
- Right heart failure & hypertrophy

» Can develop left ventricular failure & hypertrophy with severe MR

» Prone to atrial fibrillation

- Especially if the left atrium is dilated & enlarged

Causes:

» MyocardiaI infarction

» Myxomatous degeneration

- Connection tissue disorder

» Ruptured chordae tendineae or papillary muscle

- Acute mitral insufficiency!
- May need surgical repair

» Severe left heart failure

» Left ventricular hypertrophy

» Dilated cardiomyopathy

» Mitral valve prolapse

» Rheumatic heart disease

» Endocarditis

Treatment:

» If asymptomatic, medically manage

- Monitor LV function closely!

» MitraClip - mitral valve clip

- FDA approved for high surgical risk patients
- Catheter inserted via femoral vein to the right side of the heart

- Trans-atrial/septal puncture is made and catheter advanced through the mitral valve
  ▷ Monitor for signs of left to right shunting post procedure!!
  ▷ Measure oxygen saturation of the right atrium (from CVP/RAP)
  ▷ If the $ScvO_2$ is elevated, there is likely communication between the atria
  ▷ Notify the provider immediately!

- Clip(s) deployed from the underside of the mitral valve leaflets to minimize & abolish regurgitation almost immediately

» Mitral valve repair or replacement

- Can be done minimally invasive

- May opt to do the MAZE procedure for afib at the same time

- Repair is sometimes preferred
  ▷ Bonus: Long term anticoagulation is not needed!

Mitral Valve Repair or Replacement for Mitral Regurgitation Post-Op Considerations:

» The MR will cease with blood now forward flowing

» Monitor for ↑ SVR/afterload

- Treat ↑ afterload aggressively post-op!

- May need vasodilators

- ↑ SVR/afterload can lead to ↓CO

- Consider pacing if the heart rate is slower to ↑CO

» Monitor closely for right ventricular failure

- Rising CVP, increased PA pressures

» May need + inotrope (Dobutamine or Milrinone) to improve forward flow & right ventricular contractility

- In severe RV dysfunction, may need a right ventricular assist device (RVAD)

» Left ventricular failure; may need IABP for support

» If hemodynamically unstable, assess valve function with an ECHO!

» Monitor for atrial fibrillation & heart block

- May see heart block because of swelling or damage to the AV node

- Be prepared to pace!

Mitral Stenosis (MS)

» StenOsis is auscultated when the mitral valve is OPEN

» The mitral valve is Open during diastole, therefore you'll hear a:

- Diastolic murmur!

Causes:

» Rheumatic heart disease

» Endocarditis

» Left atrial myxoma

» Calcification of the valve

Signs & symptoms:

» High left atrial pressure due to the narrowed opening of the valve

  • Leads to long term left atrial enlargement & hypertrophy

» Increased pressure is back reflected to the lungs & right side of the heart

  • PA systolic pressures are often > 50 mm Hg

  • Pulmonary hypertension

  • Right ventricular failure/ hypertrophy

  • Tricuspid regurgitation (due to back flow of pressure)

  • LV function is often preserved

» Pinkish cheeks

» Fatigue

» Decreased activity tolerance

» Shortness of breath on exertion

» Pulmonary edema

» Prone to atrial fibrillation

  • Due to increased left atrial pressure & enlargement

Treatment:

» **Medical management**

  • Aimed at reducing preload & afterload

» **Surgical replacement**

» **Balloon Valvuloplasty**

  • Increases the diameter of the valve

» **Valve repair/Commissurotomy**

Mitral Valve Replacement for Mitral Stenosis
Post-Op Considerations:

» TEE is often done to assess RV & LV function

» Pulmonary hypertension will likely resolve (or PA pressures decrease)

» Will need adequate filling pressures to maintain cardiac output (right to left forward flow)

» Monitor CVP closely

  • Increasing CVP may be a sign of RV failure or compression!

  • If pre-op pulmonary hypertension, closely monitor for RV dysfunction

» May need + inotrope (Dobutamine or Milrinone) to improve forward flow & right ventricular contractility

» Will need diuretics post-op

» Monitor for new onset atrial fibrillation

» Monitor neuro assessment as there is risk of stroke!

Aortic Valve Dysfunction

The Aortic Valve

» Left heart semilunar valve

» Open during systole, closed during diastole

» 3 leaflets or cusps that open & close with pressure changes

Aortic Insufficiency/Regurgitation

» Diastolic murmur

» Results in a backflow of blood from the aortic valve to the left ventricle

» Reduced diastolic pressure with wide pulse pressure!

  • Often see high systolic with low diastolic pressures

» Increased LV compliance results in higher left ventricular AND atrial pressure

  • Leads to LV dilation & ↑ LV wall stress, ↑SVR

  • Also atrial dilation

Causes:

» Chronic hypertension

» Bicuspid aortic valve

» Aortic dissection or dilation

» Endocarditis

» Rheumatic heart disease

» Connective tissue disease

- Marfan's Syndrome

- Rheumatoid disease

» Idiopathic – means we don't know why!

Signs & symptoms:

» Slow onset & progression

- Many patients are asymptomatic for a long time!

» Dilated LV with left ventricular hypertrophy

- High pressure & volume in the left ventricle

» Can develop heart failure over time with ventricular remodeling

- Left ventricular dilation

» Monitor for mitral insufficiency over time due to volume overload

» Palpitations

» DeMusset sign – head bobbing

» Brisk carotid upstroke

» Wide pulse pressure - > 40 mm Hg (high systolic BP; low diastolic BP)

» "Water-hammer" pulse – rapid upstroke & down stroke with a shortened peak

Aortic Valve Replacement for Aortic Regurgitation
Post-Op Considerations:

» Replacement is more common than repair

» May need + inotrope (Dobutamine or Milrinone) to improve forward flow & LV emptying

- If unresponsive to inotropes, IABP for ↓CO

» Monitor SVR – Initially post-operative may be vasodilated

- May need vasopressors for decreased SVR/afterload

» Ensure adequate volume (preload), control afterload

- Also won't tolerate ↑SVR

- Will likely be hypertensive post-op (unless bleeding)

» If there is aortic root involvement, monitor for myocardial stunning/↓CO

- <u>BIG</u> SIRS response from inflammation!

» Bleeding can be an issue

» If they go into atrial fibrillation, likely will not tolerate it

- Prepare for medical or electrical cardioversion

» Monitor closely for heart block!

- Due to close proximity of the aortic valve & Bundle of His

- Edema & inflammation of the suture line

- Be prepared to epicardial pace!

- If the patient remains in heart block a few days post-op, will likely need a permanent pacemaker

Aortic Stenosis (AS)

» Sten<u>O</u>sis is auscultated when the aortic valve is <u>O</u>PEN

- The aortic valve is <u>O</u>pen during SYSTOLE, therefore the patient will have a:

- Systolic murmur!

» Most common type of valvular dysfunction

» Systolic ejection is impeded due to the narrowed opening of the calcified valve

- Increased afterload or SVR d/t to the narrowing

- Also thought to be an inflammatory component to AS

- HIGH pressure in the LV

» **Physiology:** Narrow opening → left ventricular outflow obstruction → ↑ SVR/afterload → ↓LV compliance → ↑LV pressure → ↑LV workload → diastolic dysfunction & left ventricular hypertrophy → Stiff non-compliant ventricle

» Pressure gradient between LV & aorta

- Normally the LV & aortic pressures are equal during systole
- With AS, the LV pressure increases creating a pressure gradient

» SO, these patients have LVH & diastolic dysfunction!

» Half of this patient population also has coronary artery disease

» 50%, 2-year mortality if HF develops

Causes:

» Common with elderly
  - I always jokingly say "Aortic Stenosis is earned!" (with age! ☺)
  - Usually shows up around age 70 or older
  - Calcification

» Congenital Bicuspid aortic valve
  - Usually shows up around age 40 - 60

Symptoms:

» Systolic murmur

» Angina

» Activity intolerance

» SOB, exertional dyspnea

» Syncope

» Heart failure

» Sudden cardiac death

Treatment:

» Aortic valve repair (NOT commonly done)

» Aortic valve replacement – common!
  - Median Sternotomy or small thoracotomy
  - Trans-Catheter Aortic Valve Replacement (TAVR)
    ▷ Minimally invasive

Aortic Valve Replacement for AS Post-Op Considerations:

» Manage BP & avoid hypertension

- May be challenging to control BP post-op

» Hyperdynamic left ventricle d/t drop in SVR

- The valve is open, but the left ventricular hypertrophy & stiff ventricular wall remain

- Avoid + inotropes or afterload reduction

Same as Aortic Valve Replacement for Regurgitation:

» Ensure adequate volume (preload)

- If hypotensive, likely needs volume!

» Bleeding risk!

- Assess for coagulopathy

- May develop acquired von Willebrand's with platelet dysfunction
  ▷ Prepare to administer DDAVP & platelets!

» If they go into atrial fibrillation, likely will not tolerate it

- Prepare for rate control, medical or electrical cardioversion

» Monitor closely for heart block!

- Due to close proximity of the aortic valve & Bundle of His

- Edema & inflammation on the suture line

- Be prepared to epicardial pace!

- If the patient remains in heart block a few days post-op, will need a permanent pacemaker

Transcatheter Aortic Valve Replacement (TAVR)

» Originally, FDA approved for high risk patients with aortic stenosis

- Now also low & moderate risk

- Usually performed in the Cath Lab, some in a hybrid OR

» Minimally invasive, replace the aortic valve while the heart is still beating

- Moderate procedural sedation or general anesthesia is used

» Biologic valve placed on a balloon catheter

- Guided from the femoral artery to the mid-aortic valve
  ▷ Can also access from apical or subclavian

- The balloon is then inflated & the valve deployed

- Heparinized during the procedure

Post-procedure, MONITOR:

» Femoral (or procedural) insertion site!!!!

- Vascular injury can happen

- Hematoma, bleeding

- Retro-peritoneal bleed

» Neuro assessment

- Signs of stroke or TIA

- Up to 5% incidence

» Control BP with established, tight parameters

- Typically 100 – 140 mm Hg systolic

» Atrial fibrillation

» Heart block or new left BBB

- Due to edema around the aortic valve

- Close proximity of the aortic valve to the Bundle of His!

- Be prepared to pace!

- If the patient has a pre-procedure right BBB, will likely need to be paced!

» Renal function due to IV contrast dye load

» ECHO is often done post procedure to assess for insufficiency

Tricuspid & Pulmonic Valve Dysfunction

Tricuspid valve regurgitation

» Usually secondary to right heart failure or pulmonary hypertension

» Can be congenital

Symptoms:

» RV dilation, ↑RV pressures, ↑CVP, ↑PVR (if pulmonary HTN)

» Liver congestion

» Right heart failure symptoms, peripheral edema

Treatment:

» Tricuspid valve repair

- Annuloplasty; ring in the annulus of the valve

- Valvuloplasty – if there is tricuspid stenosis

» Replacement

Tricuspid Valve Replacement for TR Post-Op Considerations:

» Monitor for RV failure!!!!

- ↑CVP → ↓CO

- Establish CVP target

» Monitor for heart block

- Potential damage to the AV node

- Can develop complete heart bloc

- Also monitor for new BBB

- Be prepared to pace!

Pulmonic Valve Dysfunction

» Is rare

» Usually secondary to congenital issues like Tetralogy of Fallot

» Monitor for right heart failure & BBB

All surgeries – valve choice:

Biologic (tissue) valve vs. Mechanical valve

Valve type:	Pros:	Cons:
Biologic (tissue)	- Does not require long-term anticoagulation	- Less durable (last ~ 10 – 20 years) - Leaflets can get stiff & calcified
Mechanical	- Lasts longer (~ 20 + years) - More durable	- Increased risk of thrombosis - Require lifelong anticoagulation with Warfarin

Infective Endocarditis (IE)

» Infection of the
endocardium or valve

» Damaged leaflets

Causes/at risk:

» Prosthetic valves

» Intra-cardiac devices
(ICD, pacemaker)

» Bacteria from other sources

» IV drug abuse (especially
tricuspid & pulmonic valve)

» At risk: Cardiac surgery,
rheumatic heart disease,
dental procedures

Symptoms:

» Stabbing, sharp pain
(worse on inspiration)

» SOB, cough

» JVD

» Fever

» Pulsus paradoxus

» Friction rub

» ST elevations on 12 Lead ECG

» Narrow pulse pressure

» Elevated WBC, ESR

» Osler's nodes

• Painful subcutaneous
lesions in the fingers

» Janeway lesions

• Painless hemorrhagic lesions
on the palms & soles

Complications of IE:

» Heart failure

» Valvular insufficiency

» Renal failure

» Stroke

» 25% risk of death

Endocarditis common organisms:

» Staphylococcus aureus
  – most common*

» Streptococcus

» Enterococcus

» Gram negative bacilli

» Fungus (i.e. candida)

Treatment:

» Administer appropriate
  antibiotics

» Usually high dose IV antibiotics

» Antibiotic duration
  usually 4 - 6 weeks

» Surgical debridement with
  valve replacement

Various cardiac assessment findings:

Pulsus paradoxus

» Decrease in systolic pressure during inspiration > 10 mm Hg caused by
  cardiac tamponade, pleural effusion, pericarditis or dehydration

Pulsus alternans

» Finding on arterial waveform
  showing alternating
  strong & weak beats.

» Indicative of left ventricular
  systolic impairment

Pericardial Rubs

» Scratching, grating,
  squeaking leather quality

» Left lower sternal border,
  leaning forward or lying
  supine in deep expiration

» High frequency

» 3 sounds are present

  • One systolic – occurs
    anywhere in systole

  • Two diastolic – occurs
    w/ ventricular stretch at
    early and late diastole

» Auscultated in MI, pericarditis, autoimmune, trauma, s/p cardiac surgery, autoimmune diseases

Overall "itis" treatment goals:

» Prevent/relieve symptoms (lean forward)

» NSAIDs (ASA or indomethacin)

» Treat infection

» Corticosteroids

» Chronic: partial pericardiectomy

• Window is created allowing fluids to drain into pleural space

Constrictive pericarditis: total pericardiectomy

You Can Do It!

Chapter 6

Thoracic Surgery & Repair of Aneurysms

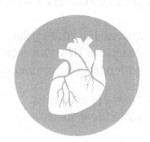

Topics covered in this chapter include:

- ▶ **Hypertension Guidelines**
  - Hypertensive Emergency
- ▶ **IV Medications used for emergent blood pressure control**
  - Beta Blockers
  - Calcium Channel Blockers
  - Nitrates
    - Nitroprusside toxicity
- ▶ **Aortic Dissection**
- ▶ **Thoracic Aortic Aneurysms (TAA)**
  - Repair of thoracic aortic aneurysm/dissection (Endografts, open repair)
  - Lower limb defects (spinal cord ischemia, paralysis)
  - Lumbar Drains
- ▶ **Abdominal Aortic Aneurysm (AAA)**
- ▶ **Ventricular aneurysm**
- ▶ **Ventricular Septal Defect (VSD)**
  - Non-congenital
  - Congenital
- ▶ **Atrial Septal Defect (ASD)**
- ▶ **Surgical treatment of Lung CA**

Hypertension Guidelines

» Updated in 2017 by the American Heart Association with tighter recommendations!

» Newer goal in most patients: < 130/80 mm Hg

» Hypertensive urgency: SBP > 180 & DBP > 120

» Hypertensive **emergency**: SBP > 180 + target organ damage

» Acute elevation associated with organ damage:

- **Kidney:** decreased blood flow, hematuria, proteinuria
- **Brain:** hypertensive encephalopathy
- **Heart:** LVH, LVF, MI
- **Eyes:** retinal hemorrhages
- **Vascular system:** vessel damage

Category	SBP		DBP
Normal	< 120	and	< 80
Elevated	120 - 129	and	< 80
Stage 1 HTN	130 - 139	or	80-89
Stage 2 HTN	≥ 140	or	≥ 90
Hypertensive urgency	> 180	and/or	> 120

Source: 2017 AHA Hypertension Guidelines

Commonly managed long term with one or more of these medications:

» ACE Inhibitor OR

» Angiotensin Receptor Blocker (ARB)

» Calcium Channel Blocker

» Thiazide diuretic

Hypertensive Emergency

Acute BP elevation associated with organ damage

» Renal: decreased blood flow, hematuria, proteinuria

» Brain: hypertensive encephalopathy, confusion

» Heart: LVH, LVF, MI

» Eyes: retinal hemorrhages

» Vascular system: vessel damage

Treatment:

» BP in both arms (r/o aneurysm, dissection or steal syndrome)

» Decrease BP by 25% in 1 - 2 hrs

» IV anti-hypertensives (vasodilators, diuretics, etc.)

- Nitroprusside (Nipride)

- Nitroglycerin (Tridil)
- Labetaolol (Trandate)
- Esmolol (Brevibloc)
- Nicardipine (Cardene)
- Cleviprex (Clevidipine)
- Fenoldopam (Corlopam)

» Consider 12 Lead ECG

IV Medications for Emergent Blood Pressure Control

Beta Blockers:

Esmolol (Brevibloc)

» Short acting beta blocker

Dosing:

» Initial dose: 250 - 500 mcg/kg IV over 1 min

» Maintenance dose: 0.05 – 0.3 mg/kg/min or 50 – 200 mcg/kg/min

Labetalol (Trandate)

» Blocks alpha, B_1 & B_2

» Negative inotropic effects, added benefit of decreasing the force of contraction to decrease myocardial workload

Dosing:

» Initial dose: 20 mg IV over 2 min

» Follow with 20 - 80 mg IV every 10 – 15 min until BP is controlled

» Maintenance dose: 2 mg/min IV continuous infusion; titrate up to 5 - 20 mg/min; not to exceed total dose of 300 mg

Metoprolol

» Beta blocker

» Dose: 5 mg IV every 2 min, up to 15 mg

Calcium Channel Blockers:

Clevidipine (Cleviprex)

» Calcium channel blocker, very short acting

» Controls influx of calcium into the cell

» Arterial vasodilator

  • Doesn't have much effect on preload (venous vasculature)

Dosing:

» 1 – 2 mg/hour IV, double every few minutes

» Maximum of 32 mg/hour IV

» Half-life is ~ 1 min

Watch out!:

» Headache

» Nausea/vomiting

» Use cautiously in ↓EF & severe aortic stenosis

» Avoid in egg & soy allergies

Nicardipine (Cardene)

» Calcium channel blocker

» Direct arterial vasodilator

• Doesn't have much effect on preload (venous vasculature)

Dosing:

» 5 – 15 mg/hr continuous infusion

» Goals: ↓BP, MAP, SVR

Watch out!:

» Hypotension

» Headache

» Nausea/vomiting

Nitrates:

Nitroglycerin (Tridil)

» Potent peripheral vasodilator

» Used to treat: angina, HF, HTN

» Dilates arterial & venous vasculature

• Mostly a preload reducer with some afterload reduction

Dosing:

» 5 mcg/min up to 200 mcg/min infusion

» Can titrate pretty quickly – every 5 to 10 minutes

Watch out!:

» Hypotension, bradycardia, dizziness, hypovolemia, headache, reflexive tachycardia, N/V

» In some people NTG doesn't have much effect on the BP, develop tolerance

» Do not use in hypotension, hypovolemia, aortic stenosis, ICP issues, constrictive pericarditis

Nitroprusside (Nipride)

» Antihypertensive of
   nitrate origin

» Arteriolar & venous vasodilation

» **Potent vasodilator!
   Reduces afterload/SVR!

» *Monitor thiocyanate
   level for toxicity!

Dosing:

» 0.5 – 8 mcg/kg/min continuous infusion

Watch out!:

» Hypotension

  • Assess BP every 1 - 2 min
    until BP is stabilized

  • Arterial line preferred

» Hypoxia

  • From intrapulmonary shunting

» Increased HR

  • Due to stimulation of
    baroreceptors

» Thiocyanate toxicity

  • Especially with > 72 hours of use

  • Monitor serum thiocyanate levels

  • Methemoglobinemia -
    hemoglobin can get converted

Nitroprusside Toxicity

» Thiocyanate toxicity occurs infrequently

Clinical signs:

» Vasodilation resulting in
   hypotension &/or dysrhythmias

» Tinnitus, altered mental status
   changes, nausea, abdominal pain

» Coma, metabolic acidosis,
   or respiratory arrest

» In rare cases,
   Methemoglobinemia can occur;
   if levels reach >15%, can cause
   symptomatic cellular hypoxia

» Toxicity risk =

  • Prolonged administration

  • Renal &/or liver dysfunction

Nitroprusside Toxicity Treatment

» Cyanide toxicity: treat with 100% oxygen to maximize oxygen availability

» Administer sodium thiosulfate (150 mg/kg over 15 min) or 3% sodium nitrate (5 mg/kg over 5 min)

• Oxidizes hemoglobin to methemoglobin, or by limiting the administration of nitroprusside

» Methemoglobinemia: from excessive doses of sodium nitroprusside –

• Methylene blue (1 – 2 mg/kg of a 1% solution over 5 min)

• Reduces methemoglobin to hemoglobin

Other:

Fenoldopam (Corlopam)

Dosing:

» Initiate dosing at 0.01 - 0.3 mcg/kg/min by IV infusion

» Titrate by 0.05 - 0.1 mcg/kg/min every 15 min or longer until target blood pressure reached

• Up to 1.6 mcg/kg/min used in clinical trials

» May continue maintenance infusion for up to 48 hours

» Pharmacokinetics

• Half-Life: 5 min

• Duration: 1 - 4 hour post infusion

• Onset: 10 min, max effect: 30 - 120 min

Monitor: Angina, dysrhythmias, dizziness, flushing, heart failure, hypotension, tachycardia, headache, N/V, creatinine level (can increase)

» Mechanism of Action:

• D1-dopamine receptor agonist: rapid-acting vasodilator

• Decreases peripheral resistance

• Increases renal blood flow; has minimal adrenergic effects

• Also diuretic, natriuretic

Aortic Dissection & Aortic Aneurysms

» Aortic dissection

» Thoracic (TAA)

» Abdominal (AAA)

General thoughts on aneurysms & dissection:

Major risk factors:

» Hypertension & smoking are major risk factors

» Smoking is the biggest modifiable risk factor

» Family history

» Advanced age

• Average is 70 years old

• Males age 60s – 80s (typical)

» Bicuspid aortic valve

» Cocaine or Meth abuse

» Trauma – MVC with acceleration/deceleration forces

» Connective tissue disorders

• Marfan's Syndrome

» Atherosclerosis

» Weight lifting

» Strain on the vessel wall

Goal: Prevent rupture or dissection

Aortic Dissection:

» Medical emergency!!!!

• Rupture = ~ 90% mortality!!!!

» Tear in the intimal lining of the aortic vessel wall

» Causes a split between the intimal & middle layer of the aorta

» Graded as Stanford System Type A or Type B

» Type A: Ascending aorta

• Can extend from aortic arch to the left ventricle

• Most dissections are Type A dissection

• Will require surgery!

» Type B: Descending aorta/ any other dissection

- Starts in the descending aorta

» Can extend past the aortic arch to the abdomen

- Less life threatening

- May complain of epigastric, scapular or flank pain

- May also have referred pain (not in the location of the aneurysm)

- Often associated with atherosclerosis

- Usually medically managed

- BP control: beta blockers & vasodilators

- Control pain

- Long term: May need surgery or endovascular stenting

Type A Aortic Dissection Symptoms:

» Mimics other conditions – i.e. myocardial infarction

» Acute onset of SEVERE pain!

- Abrupt onset, "stabbing", "ripping", "tearing" sharp pain

- Between the scapula

» Dyspnea

» Raspy voice

» Syncope

» Weakness or paralysis on one side of the body

» Altered mental status

» BP difference of 25 mm Hg or greater between left & right arm

General treatment goals:

» Go to the OR immediately!!!

» Surgical repair – synthetic grafting to replace the dissected area

» Immediate priority: Heart rate, blood pressure & pain control!

- IV opiates commonly used

» Want to provide negative inotropy to reduce the force of myocardial contraction

- "Anti-Impulse Therapy"

- First line: Beta blockers***
  ▷ Labetalol, esmolol
  ▷ Block SNS/catecholamine release

- Second choice (if BB contraindicated): Calcium channel blocker

- FYI – Contraindications to beta blockers: severe asthma, COPD, severe bradycardia, heart block, severe systolic heart failure

» Heart rate control

- Goal heart rate < 60 bpm

- Beta blockers*** or calcium channel blocker (if can't take a BB)

- Labetalol commonly used for HR & BP control

» Assess BP: tight control

- Generally target SBP < 120 mm Hg, MAP 65 – 75 mm Hg; lowest possible to perfuse organs!
- Nicardipine is often used
- If hypotensive, start a vasopressor
- Assess fluid status – consider volume
- Prepare for transfusion

» Intra-Aortic Balloon Counterpulsation (IABC/IABP) is contraindicated!

» Diagnosis is made most often by CT scan

- Also consider ultrasound & MRI
- Chest radiograph – may see wide mediastinum
- TEE to assess aortic valve & LV function
- 12 Lead ECG

Post-operative, monitor for complications:

» Tamponade

» Intramural thrombus

» Aortic insufficiency

» Myocardial infarction

- Low coronary perfusion

» Acute Kidney Injury (AKI)

» Limb ischemia

Thoracic Aortic Aneurysm

» Dilatation of the aorta > 50% of its normal diameter

» Larger diameter & enlargement weakens the vessel wall over time

- Often progress slowly

Thoracic Aortic Aneurysm (TAA) Pre-Operative:

» Patients will often describe "ripping" or "stabbing" chest pain radiating to the back

» Immediate goal is to prevent rupture of the aneurysm!

» At risk for aortic insufficiency (AI)

- An ECHO or TEE is often done to assess for AI
- Diastolic murmur
- May have wide pulse pressure (> 40 mm Hg)

Treatment:

» Surgery

- TAAA: Thoraco-abdominal aortic aneurysm

- TEVAR: Thoracic endovascular aortic repair

- Bentall Procedure: Aortic Valve, ascending aorta & root replacement

» Sternotomy often with Circulatory Arrest & deep hypothermia

- Especially if the aortic root or valve needs to be replaced

- Deep hypothermia for neuro protection

- Sometimes as low as 14 - 18°C, moderate range 28°C

- Will re-warm slowly in the OR using CPB circuit

Post-Operative Considerations from Surgical Repair of TAA:

» Bleeding!!!!

- May be more prone to bleeding & coagulopathy from hypothermia

- Often need lots of blood products

- Coagulopathy: May need FFP, PCC (KCentra), DDAVP, cryoprecipitate

- RBCs – don't forget to replace calcium!

- Long CPB times

» Major post-operative concern is Paraplegia!

- Aorta cross-clamping can lead to spinal cord ischemia/infarction

- TAAA incidence 8 – 28%

- TEVAR 4 – 7%

- Assess motor function as soon as anesthesia wears off & patient starts to wake up

  ▷ Assessment: Can the patient bend their knee & lift their leg?

  ▷ Lower extremity sensation, weakness, numbness?

- Goal: Augment spinal cord perfusion

- Optimize blood pressure, AVOID hypotension!!!!

- Targets need to be individualized, but in general keep MAP > 80 mm Hg

- Lumbar drains used to optimize spinal cord perfusion

- Spinal cord perfusion pressure (PP):

  ▷ MAP – Lumbar CSF pressure = Spinal cord PP

  ▷ Keep Spinal cord PP > 70 mm Hg

    - Use vasopressors if needed

▷ Goal CSF pressure <
10 – 12 mm Hg

▷ CSF drain left in for 2 – 3 days

▷ AVOID rapid drainage of CSF!!!

▷ If the drain isn't functional,
it needs to be replaced!

» Pain control

» Renal function

» Swallow reflex may be impaired

• Swallow evaluation if difficulties

Abdominal Aortic Aneurysm (AAA)

» Aneurysm is usually located
below the renal arteries

» Pulsation in the abdomen

» Tightly control blood pressure!

» Surgical repair

Signs of rupture:

» Pain

• Ischemia to areas below
the aneurysm

• Often imitates other medical
issues (i.e. kidney stones,
MI, gall stones, etc.)

» Hypotension

» Tachycardia

» Shock

» Rupture – 90% mortality!!!!!

Post-Operative Surgical Repair of AAA:

» BP control

» Pain management

» Wean from ventilator

» Monitor chest tube output

» Closely monitor urine output

• May see increased BUN
& creatinine due to
aortic cross-clamp

» Monitor for bleeding

» Extremity movement

» Other post-op practices

Ventricular Aneurysm

» Bulge or 'pocketing' of the wall or lining of a vessel in the left ventricle

* Swells into a "bubble" of blood
* Can form in the blood vessels at the base of the septum, or within the aorta
* The aneurysm can have a clot within it

» Can happen after a myocardial infarction – usually develop slowly

» Patient may present with heart failure, ↓CO/SV or ventricular arrhythmias

Symptoms:

» May see ST elevation on 12 Lead ECG

» Depending on the size, it may impede blood flow to the body

» Clots can form within the aneurysm

» Monitor for signs of embolism:

* CVA symptoms
* Limb ischemia

Diagnosis:

» ECHO

* Assess for mitral insufficiency

» Pre-operative cardiac catheterization

Treatment:

» They may not need treatment

* Anticoagulation to prevent thrombus formation
* ACE Inhibitors may be preventative after MI

» Surgery – ventricular reduction & removal of scar tissue

» Post-operative may need support with + inotropes or IABP

Ventricular Septal Defect/Rupture

Non-Congenital

» Can form days to weeks following a septal wall MI

» Disruption of the septal wall that results in left to right shunting of blood

Symptoms:

» Acute SOB

» S3 heart sound

» Crackles

» Holosystolic murmur

» PA catheter insertion:

- Falsely elevated C.O. on PA Cath because C.O. reading is derived from the right ventricle (left to right shunting)

- Increased SvO_2 due to left to right shunting
  ▷ Oxygen rich blood shunts left to right

- Large "v" waves on CVP waveform

» Monitor for Complete Heart Block or BBB

» Hypotension

» Pulmonary hypertension

Diagnostics:

» ECHO

- May see functional mitral valve regurgitation

- Assess tricuspid valve

Treatment:

» May need + inotropes for support

» IABP for support

» Surgical repair with septal grafting

» Will require CPB

Congenital Ventricular Septal Defect

» Often surgically
repaired as a baby

» Usually closes before puberty

» As an adult increased risk of
valve dysfunction & endocarditis

» If symptomatic, plan
for surgical repair

Atrial Septal Defect (ASD)

» Most common congenital
defect in adults

Symptoms:

» SOB, fatigue

» May have pulmonary
hypertension

» Murmur

» Stroke may be the first symptom
for some people (this happened
with one of my friends
when she was pregnant)

» Atrial fibrillation

Diagnosis:

» ECHO

» TEE with bubble study

• Often see left to right shunting

• Assess the right side of the heart

▷ Right ventricular enlargement
▷ Pulmonary HTN
▷ Tricuspid regurg

• May see Patent Foramen
Ovale (PFO)
▷ Right to left shunting

Treatment:

» Surgical or percutaneous closure

» Big Stroke risk!!!!

Lung Cancer

» Patients often present with c/o cough, shortness of breath, hemoptysis, fatigue, weight loss

» Diagnosed usually by chest radiograph → CT scan → biopsy

3 common types of surgery:

» Wedge resection

- Small wedge of lung tissue removed

» Lobectomy

- A lobe of the lung is removed

» Pneumonectomy

- Entire lung removed from one side

- May also remove lymph nodes

Post-Operative concerns from Lung Cancer Surgery

Fluids

» DO NOT FLUID OVERLOAD!!!!

» In the first 24 hours, usually give < 20 ml/kg TOTAL fluid

» Lower hemoglobin may be OK in this population

» Usually don't transfuse unless the Hgb < 7g/dL & they are symptomatic

» Monitor for pulmonary edema

- More common with right pneumonectomy

- Right pneumonectomy patients have challenges
  ▷ The right carries > 50% of lung volume & vasculature

Pain

» Big issue!!!!

» Pain can last for months after surgery

» After OR, use a multi-modal approach to management

- Epidural or nerve blocks

- NSAIDs, acetaminophen, ketamine

- Gabapentin

Chest tubes

» Will have a prolonged air leak

- Remain in place until the air leak has resolved

» Often placed to water seal

» For pneumonectomy: NEVER place CT to suction!

- May see mediastinal shift

» If there is sudden bleeding, contact the provider STAT!

- Will need to return to surgery
- Assess for coagulopathy

Other post-operative concerns:

Atelectasis!!!

» Cough, deep breath, incentive spirometry

» Chest PT if needed

» Early mobility is a MUST!

Positioning:

» Position operative lung DOWN, good lung UP!!!

- Promotes fluid filling of the removed lung

» Out of bed as much as possible

» DVT prophylaxis

Cardiovascular events

» Monitor for cardiac ischemia

» Atrial fibrillation in up to 30% of patients!

- If afib, don't usually use Amiodarone for pneumonectomy due to pulmonary toxicity side effects

- Use beta blockers, Diltiazem
- If lobectomy can use BB, Dilt or Amio

You Can Do It!

Chapter 7

Bleeding, Coagulopathies & Anticoagulation

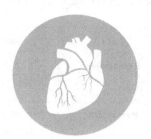

Topics covered in this chapter include:

▶ Hematology Review

- Anemia
- Thrombocytopenia

▶ Bleeding & Reversal Agents

- Heparin rebound
- Protamine use & reactions
- Vitamin K

▶ Alternative options to control bleeding

- Cryoprecipitate
- Prothrombin Complex Concentrate (PCC)
- Tranexamic acid (TXA)
- Aminocaproic Acid (Amicar)

▶ von Willebrand Disease

▶ Anticoagulation

- Warfarin
- Heparin
- LMW Heparin
- Direct Oral Anticoagulation (DOAC)

▶ Heparin Induced thrombocytopenia (HIT)

Hematology Review

Lab:	Normal:	Treat if:	Treat with:
Hemoglobin	12 – 16 g/dL Up to 17.5 g/dL in men	< 7.0 – 8.0 g/dL, higher threshold if actively bleeding	PRBCs, assess coags
Hematocrit	35 – 45% Up to 50% in men	< 21%, higher threshold if actively bleeding	PRBCs, assess coags
Platelets	150 – 450,000 per microliter	It depends, especially if the patient has impaired platelet function, < 75 – 100K	Platelets
Fibrinogen	150 – 400 mg/dL	< 100 – 150 & actively bleeding	Cryoprecipitate
PT/INR	11 – 13.5 seconds 0.8 – 1.1 INR	INR > 1.5, bleeding or oozy with elevation	FFP, Vitamin K, PCC (Kcentra) DDAVP/Desmopressin
PTT	25 – 38 seconds	Bleeding or oozy with elevation	Protamine
ACT	70 – 120 seconds	Bleeding or oozy with elevation	Protamine

Anemia

» Defined Hgb < 12 g/dL

» Reasons for anemia:

- Obvious...in cardiac surgery is bleeding!

- Frequent phlebotomy

- Systemic inflammation from CPB

- ↓ RBC production

- Iron &/or vitamin B12 deficiency

- Chronic illness

» RBC production is regulated by erythropoietin

» Transfusion threshold.... It depends!!!

» Generally Hemoglobin <
7 g/dL, Hematocrit < 21%
if the patient is stable

  • Hint: Hemoglobin level
  multiplied by 3 gives you
  a hematocrit level

• If a patient is actively bleeding,
please don't wait until the
Hgb is < 7 to transfuse!

• In actively bleeding
patients the transfusion
threshold is much higher

n general...

» Anemia is tolerated as long as
intravascular volume is adequate

» Hemoglobin & Hematocrit
tell you very little about
oxygen utilization!

• SvO$_2$/ScvO$_2$ give a better
idea of how the patient
is utilizing oxygen

• All they tell you is how many
cells the patient has

latelets

» Normal 150,000 – 450,000/uL

» Also called thrombocytes
d/t their role in clotting

» ~65% of platelets circulate in
blood, ~35% stored in spleen

» Platelet transfusion reactions
are the most common

Coagulopathies & Platelet Disorders

In thrombocytopenia, either:

» Not enough platelets or there is
impaired function of the platelet

» Life span of a platelet is 10 days

» Any endothelial damage causes
platelets to adhere to collagen

Platelet Transfusions

» When whole blood is donated, platelets get separated with leukocytes

- Increased incidence of fever with platelet transfusion d/t leukocytes

» Banked platelets are usually pooled

» Store banked platelets up to 7 days

» Viability decreases after 3 days

» Infusion of platelets

- 30,000/uL rise

» See increase 1 hour after transfusion, lasts 8 days

If not seeing an increase in the platelet count with a transfusion consider:

» Leukocyte reduced transfusion

» ABO compatibility

Thrombocytopenia

» Platelet count < 150,000 /uL

» The body can form platelet plugs until the platelet count is about 100,000 /uL

» Without a structural lesion, we can tolerate platelet count ~ 5,000 /uL as long as there is no major bleeding!

» In ICUs, the incidence of thrombocytopenia is up to 35%

» Causes of thrombocytopenia:

- Cardiopulmonary bypass
- Cardiac assist devices
  ▷ IABP
  ▷ Impella
  ▷ VAD
- Heparin Induced Thrombocytopenia (HIT)
- Sepsis - Phagocytosis of platelets by macrophages
- DIC
- Inflammation

Bleeding & Reversal Agents

General thoughts, in the setting of bleeding:

» About 25 – 30% of Cardiac Surgery patients will require a transfusion

» Warfarin is usually held for 4 days pre-operative

» Clopidogrel is usually held 5 – 7 days pre-operative

» Figure out why the patient is bleeding:

- Surgical bleed

- Suture lines

- Impaired or dysfunctional platelets

- Acquired von Willebrand disease

- Inadequate Heparin reversal

- Heparin rebound

- Residual heparin or warfarin

- Depleting coagulation factors?

» Make sure the patient's temperature is normal

- Hypothermia can exacerbate bleeding

» If bleeding from chest tubes, consider replacing chest tube output 1 ml:1 ml with blood

» If the hemoglobin & hematocrit are low, transfuse:

- PRBCs (I know, a big no duh!)

- Remember PRBCs don't do anything to stop bleeding!

- When transfusing blood, anticipate to replace calcium & possibly FFP

  ▷ Citrate is a preservative added to banked blood – it leaches calcium

  ▷ Follow ionized calcium

» If the platelet count is low, transfuse:

- Platelets (I know, another big no duh!)

» If the PT/INR is elevated, use:

- Fresh Frozen Plasma (FFP), Vitamin K or Prothrombin Complex Concentrate (PCC)/Kcentra

» If the PTT is elevated, use:

- Protamine

» If the fibrinogen is low, use:

- Cryoprecipitate

» **Remember:** any agent used to stop bleeding, promotes clotting & may cause THROMBOSIS!

Heparin Rebound

» Anti-coagulant activity & bleeding observed post-operatively after Protamine given for intra-op Heparin neutralization

» See with patients who require Cardiopulmonary Bypass

» Usually see 1 to 6 hours post-op

Treatment:

» Administer Protamine

» Extended post-op administration of Protamine

• Protamine infusion 25 mg/hr

• Give if ACT > 120 seconds

Protamine sulfate for Heparin reversal

» In general, we give 25 – 50 mg IV

» Heparin: 1 – 1.5 mg/100 units of Heparin

  • Do not exceed 50 mg

» Dalteparin: 1 mg/100 units of Dalteparin administered

» Enoxaparin: 1 mg/mg of enoxaparin if enoxaparin given within 8 hours

Protamine Safety & Reactions:

» Never give more than 50 mg over 10 minutes

  • Give slowly!!!!

» Monitor for reactions:

  • Bradycardia

  • Hypotension

  • Nausea/vomiting

• Anaphylaxis – Shortness of breath & airway issues

  ▷ Polypeptide isolated from salmon sperm (fish allergy)

  ▷ Avoid in men that have had a vasectomy

  ▷ Histamine release that can cause vasodilation → ↓SVR & BP, treat with vasopressor!

  ▷ Other physical signs: tachycardia, flushing, bronchospasm, dyspnea

- Anaphylaxis treatment:
  - ▷ Epinephrine 0.3 mg IM (blocks inflammatory mediators)
- Histamine blockers: H1 – Diphenhydramine 25 – 50 mg, H2 – Pepcid or Zantac
- May consider steroids

- Interactions:
  - ▷ **Use caution if receiving NPH insulin, it is protamine based
  - ▷ PCN or Cephalosporins
- Remember, it promotes clotting, so may cause thrombosis!

Coumadin Reversal:

Vitamin K (phytonadione) Dosing non-emergent:

» 2.5 –5 mg PO

» 1 – 2.5 mg IV <u>SLOWLY</u> over an hour

» Will see INR drop within 8 – 12 hours

Serious or life threatening bleeding:

» Vitamin K 10 mg IV SLOWLY – never give IV push!

» Fresh Frozen Plasma (FFP)

» Prothrombin Complex Concentrate (PCC) KCentra®

» NovoSeven – recombinant factor seven

- Stimulates thrombin generation

Alternative options to control bleeding:

Cryoprecipitate

» Goal: Fibrinogen > 100 mg/dL

» Each bag contains 200 – 250 mg of fibrinogen

» Will increase fibrinogen by 6 – 8 mg/dL

Prothrombin Complex Concentrate (PCC)

» Reverses the effects of warfarin & other vitamin K antagonists

» Major benefit – concentrated, so don't have to administer large volumes

» Contraindicated in HIT & DIC

   • Contains Heparin

» Used for significant bleeding when INR > 8.0 (lower for some patients)

» Kcentra® contains factors II, VII, IX & X

» Factor IX complex contains II, IX & X

» Sometimes factor VII or Protein C

Anti-Fibrinolytic Agents

Tranexamic Acid (TXA)

» AKA Lysteda, Cyklokapron

» Anti-fibrinolytic

» Promotes clotting by slowing down the breakdown of blood clots

Dosing:

» 10 – 15 mg/kg (~ 1 Gram) IV over 20 min, then

» 1 mg/kg/hour via infusion for 6 – 10 hours

» Reduce dosing for renal impairment

» Remember, it promotes clotting, so may cause thrombosis!

Aminocaproic Acid (Amicar)

» Used to control bleeding – "Anti-fibrinolytic"

» Remember, it promotes clotting, so may cause thrombosis!

Dosing:

» Initial: 4 - 5 g IV/PO during 1st hour, THEN 1 - 1.25 g PO q 1 hour

» OR, Continuous IV infusion at 1 g/hour

» Continue for 8 hours or until bleeding controlled, not to exceed 30 g/day

Mechanism of Action:

» Inhibits plasminogen binding to fibrin & subsequent conversion to plasmin, which in turn inhibits fibrinolysis

» Exhibits anti-plasmin activity

Pharmacokinetics:

» Onset: 1 - 2 hours

» Duration: 3 - 4 hours (after 1 dose)

» Half-life: 2 hours

von Willebrand Disease

» Genetic clotting disorder

» Many people don't know they have it

» Deficiency in von Willebrand Factor (vWF)

• Needed for platelet adhesion

• Platelet Dysfunction

» Type 1 von Willebrand

• Bleeding treatment: Desmopressin (DDAVP), recombinant von Willebrand factor (rVWF) (Vonvendi), von Willebrand factor/factor VIII (vWF/FVIII) concentrates & platelets

• Desmopressin (DDAVP)
  ▷ 0.3 – 0.4 mcg/kg IV over 30 min
    - Can cause hypotension if given too quickly
  ▷ Improves platelet function & aggregation
  ▷ Stimulates release of vWF from platelets

▷ Monitor for water retention & dilutional hyponatremia

- FYI – doesn't have vasopressor qualities like Vasopressin

▷ May need to transfuse platelets with DDAVP! Need to have platelets for it to work!

» Type 2 von Willebrand

• Desmopressin (DDAVP) may not work for vWD Type 2

• Can do a trial administration to assess if it works

» Type 3 von Willebrand

• Will NOT be responsive to Desmopressin

• Administer recombinant von Willebrand Factor (rvWF) with or without FVIII

» Bleeding considerations:

• PRBCs, platelets (esp. if platelet-type vWD)

FYI - Review

Anticoagulation

Coumadin (Warfarin)

» Acts on extrinsic & common coagulation pathways

» Monitor PT/INR

» Therapeutic goal INR 2 – 3x baseline

• DVT Prophylaxis

• PE Prophylaxis/treatment

• Atrial fibrillation

» Therapeutic goal INR 2.5 – 3.5x baseline

• Mechanical prosthetic valves

» Reversal: Vitamin K or FFP

Heparin (unfractionated)

» Heparin is used during Cardiopulmonary Bypass (CPB) to prevent clotting

» Acts on intrinsic & common coagulation pathways

» Monitor aPTT

» Can also monitor Factor Xa

» Normal 25 – 38 seconds

» For sheath removal, can also monitor ACT

- Therapeutic ACT 300 – 350 seconds

» Discontinue sheath when ACT < 150 seconds

» Reversal: Protamine sulfate

Low Molecular Weight Heparin vs. Unfractionated Heparin

Benefits of LMWH:

» Less incidence of HIT

» No need to monitor aPTT

» Longer half-life

- 4 – 6 hours vs. 1 – 2 hours

» More predictable d/t bioavailability

- 90% bioavailable vs. 30%

Direct Oral Anticoagulation (DOAC) – FYI only				
Drug:	Works on:	Half-life:	FDA approval:	Reversal:
Dabigatran (Pradaxa)	DTI, anti-factor IIa	12 – 17 hours	Non-Valvular afib, VTE Prophylaxis	Praxbind (idarucizumab)
Rivaroxaban (Xarelto)	Factor Xa inhibitor	7 – 11 hours	Non-Valvular afib, VTE prevention	Andexxa (Andexanet alfa)
Apixaban (Eliquis)	Factor Xa inhibitor	12 hours	Venous thromboembolic events	Andexxa (Andexanet alfa)
Edoxaban (Lixiana)	Factor Xa inhibitor	10 – 14 hours	VTE Prophylaxis after ortho surgery, stroke prevention	None available
Betrixaban (Bevyxxa)	Factor Xa inhibitor		VTE, DVT/PE (hospitalized patients)	None available

Heparin Induced Thrombocytopenia (HIT)

» Platelet count drops by ≥ 50% from BASELINE within 5 – 10 days of exposure to Heparin

» May develop more quickly if previous exposure to Heparin

» Often Cardiac Surgery patients will not develop HIT until ≥ 5 days post-operative from CPB Heparin exposure

» Erythematous lesions around SQ Heparin injection sites

» 25% of patients develop systemic reaction

  • Fever

  • Chills

  • Tachypnea

  • Tachycardia

» **Major Complication: Thrombosis

  • DVT of lower extremity

  • DVT of upper extremity

  • Pulmonary embolus

  • Arterial Thrombosis

  • AMI & Stroke

» Risk is greater with unfractionated Heparin (UFH)

» Even low doses & heparin flushes!!!

» Don't forget: Heparin coated catheters!!!

Diagnosis of HIT:

» Clinical exposure to Heparin

» Thrombocytopenia

» Symptomatic thrombosis

» IgG Antibodies to Heparin

  • Platelet Factor 4 complex

  • IgG with Reflex to Serotonin Release Assay

» Clinical picture + assay for diagnosis

2 Types of HIT:

Type 1 HIT:

» 1st - 2 days after exposure to heparin, platelet count normalizes with continued heparin therapy

» Non-immune disorder that results from the direct effect of heparin on platelet activation

Type 2 HIT:

» More serious

» Immune-mediated disorder that typically occurs 4-10 days after exposure to heparin

» Life & limb-threatening thrombotic complications

Treatment of HIT:

» Discontinue all forms of Heparin!!!

» Anticoagulation using Direct Thrombin Inhibitors:

» Bivalirudin

- Initial: 0.15 - 0.2 mg/kg/hr IV

- Monitor PTT, no effect on INR

- Adjust to aPTT 1.5 - 2.5 times baseline value

- Half-life is 25 min

- Renal adjustments are necessary

» Argatroban

- Cleared by the liver

- 2 mcg/kg/min – Max 10 mcg/kg/min

- Monitor PTT, but it does have an effect on INR

- PTT 1.5 – 3 x baseline value, not to exceed 100 seconds

- Half-life is 50 min

» Long term anticoagulation with Coumadin

» HOWEVER, do not use during the active phase of HIT

- Increased risk of tissue necrosis & limb gangrene

» Heparin antibodies last > 100 days after exposure

» Do not reintroduce Heparin as long as antibodies persist!

You Can Do It!

Chapter 8

Electrical Issues

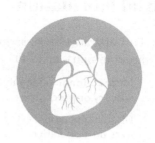

Topics covered in this chapter include:

- ► Atrial Fibrillation
- ► Atrial ECG post-operative
- ► MAZE Procedure
- ► Atrial Flutter
- ► Rate control & anti-dysrhythmic medications
- ► Tachyarrhythmias
- ► Bradyarrhythmias & Heart Blocks
- ► Emergent pacing options

Atrial Fibrillation

» Post-operative atrial arrhythmias are common – up to 40 – 60%

  • More common after valvular surgery or procedures

  • Often happens at 2 – 4 days post-operative

  • PACs are a warning sign!

  • Usually convert back to sinus rhythm within 6 – 8 weeks post-op

  • Increases hospital length of stay

» Known as the "neuro rhythm" or "stroke rhythm" because of the embolic stroke incidence

» When patients are in afib, blood becomes stagnant especially in the left atrial appendage and can coagulate = BIG STROKE risk!!!!

» This is why many CT surgeons often do left atrial appendage closures with CABG

» Atrial muscle fibers depolarizing erratically

  • Multi-focal stimuli in the atria

  • The AV node is irregularly stimulated

  • AV node is intermittently refractory to the impulses

  • Intermittent signals make it to the ventricles

  • Lose atrial kick - ↓ in C.O. by up to 25%

  • Better tolerated with normal heart function

» Ventricular rate 100 – 200 bpm

» Long term can develop atrial enlargement

» Anti-coagulation if > 24 hours

Risk factors for developing post-operative atrial fibrillation & atrial flutter

» ↑ age

» Valvular disease

» MI/CAD

» Rheumatic Heart Disease

» Pre-operative left atrial enlargement

  • > 4.5 cm

» LV diastolic dysfunction

» Left ventricular hypertrophy

» Dilated right atrium &/ or right ventricle

» Pre-op beta blocker withdrawal

» Electrolyte imbalances – specifically hypomagnesemia

» Bleeding

» Catecholamine infusions

» Inflammation

» Poor intra-operative myocardial protection

» Cardioplegia solution

Management of atrial fibrillation post-operative:

» You need to decide to rate vs. rhythm control

• Medical/electrical conversion or both

» In chronic afib, would never want to convert unless verified via TEE there is no thrombus present

» Thrombus most often form in the left atrium & left atrial appendage

» Anticoagulation is necessary, especially if in afib > 24 - 48°

Medication options:

» Beta blockers* (Ex. Esmolol, metoprolol)

• There are some data supporting pre-op afib prophylaxis with BB

• Often administered the morning of surgery

• Can administer BB with Mg^{++} IV usually with good effect!

» Rate control options: BB, CCB or Amio

» Synchronized cardioversion if new & unstable

» Amiodarone – safer to use with reduced ejection fraction

» Calcium channel blockers* (Ex. diltiazem)

• *Use cautiously in patients with reduced EF

• Provides rate control

» Sotalol

• Effective in preventing afib

• Contraindicated in heart failure

» Digoxin

» Always know the patient's electrolyte levels when treating arrhythmias!

- Replace electrolytes to a normal level!

• Pay attention to potassium & magnesium!

» Often rate control & anticoagulated since it usually resolves 6 – 8 weeks post-op

Atrial ECG:

» Useful for differentiating origin of suspect atrial & junctional arrhythmias

» Assists in defining the nature of an AV block by amplifying atrial activity

» Allows you to evaluate atrial activity in relationship to ventricular activity

How to:

» 12 Lead ECG: connect atrial wires to leads V1 & V2

» Bedside ECG monitor: Connect atrial wires to right & left arm leads; all other leads stay the same

MAZE Procedure

» There are multiple variations of the procedure

- Commonly you'll hear about the "Mini-MAZE" which can be performed endoscopically

» Long term treatment of chronic atrial fibrillation

» The success rate is upwards of 80 – 90%!

» Surgical incisions made to left &/or right atria in a maze-like pattern to form scar tissue

- Scar tissue doesn't conduct erratic impulses

- Blocks abnormal pathways & irregular electrical activity

- Creating a new route for conduction

» Most procedures are performed minimally invasive

  • Can also perform open chest procedure

» Many times the left atrial appendage will also be removed or closed with the MAZE procedure

Post-procedure:

» May still be in afib with resolution over time

» Continue antiarrhythmic medications

» Diuretics usually administered d/t swelling

» Start/resume anticoagulation – usually warfarin (Coumadin)

Atrial Flutter – FYI

» Atrial rates 240 – 400 beats/ min, ventricular rates can vary

» AV node conduction block

» Symptoms: Syncope, palpitations, fatigue, exercise intolerance, SOB

» ~ 60% have underlying CAD

  • Sequelae of open heart surgery

» Catheter ablation is superior (long term) to rate & rhythm control

  • TTE – preferred method for evaluating atrial flutter

  • TEE – Best for viewing left atrium for thrombus

Atrial Overdrive Pacing:

» Atrial Overdrive Pace

  • Used in attempt to terminate:
    ▷ Atrial flutter

» Can be performed in patients with atrial epicardial pacing wires

» Post open heart surgery

» Pace the atria at rates over 300 – 400 bpm

  • Basically pace faster than the flutter rate

  • May allow for the sinus node to take over

  • For safety, we usually disconnect the ventricular wires (hopefully it's obvious why! ☺)

Medications:

Amiodarone

» Used to treat atrial or ventricular arrhythmias

» Effects mostly on K^+ channels in myocardial cells

» Atrial arrhythmias – dose 150 mg over 10 min IV, then 1 mg/min x 6 hours, then 0.5 mg/min x 18 hours

- Use a filter
- Transition to PO dosing after IV is complete

» Adverse effects - Monitor QTc interval, as it will prolong

» Hypotension, bradycardia, heart block, increased liver enzymes (all rare)

» Toxicity: pulmonary fibrosis, neuro or hepatic injury, thyroid dysfunction

» Has a looooooooooong half-life of about 58 days!!!! Whoa!

Beta Blockers

General for BB:

» Watch out! for:

- Bradycardia

- Hypotension
- Heart block
- Wheezing/broncho-constriction

Metoprolol (Lopressor)

» Selectively blocks $beta_1$ receptors

» Effects: reduces HR, prolongs AV node conduction, suppresses renin secretion

» Negative inotrope, so decreases contractility & C.O.

» Dose: 5 mg every 5 min up to about 15 mg

» Adverse effects: Bradycardia, hypotension, heart failure, hypoglycemia

» Use with caution in asthmatic patients!

Esmolol (Brevibloc)

» Selectively blocks beta$_1$ receptors

» Used to treat SVT, rate control for Afib & flutter, HTN

» Dose: Bolus 500 mcg/ kg (over 1 min),

  • Then start infusion at 25 – 50 mcg/kg/min

  • Increase by 50 mcg/kg/ min every 5 – 10 min

• Maximum is about 200 mcg/kg/min infusion

» Onset 1 – 2 min

» Short half-life (< 10 min), so if patient develops side effects, shut it off

» Adverse effects: Hypotension, bradycardia, heart block, heart failure, bronchospasm

Diltiazem (Cardizem)

» Calcium channel blocker

» Decreases AV node conduction & causes vasodilation

» Negative chronotropic effects (potent) and mild negative inotropic effects

» Used in afib & flutter and PSVT

» Also used to treat angina, HTN

» Dose: Push 5 – 20 mg IV

  • Then start infusion 5 – 15 mg/hr

  • Titrate to HR & BP

» Can transition to PO Dilt; stop infusion after 1st dose

» Half-life is 3 – 4.5 hours

» Adverse effects: Hypotension, 2nd or 3rd degree AV block, bradycardia, asystole, heart failure, N/V

Digoxin (Lanoxin)

» Positive inotrope (increases contractility), increases calcium influx into cells

» Slows AV node conduction

» Used in Afib, flutter & PSVT (not first line, use BB or CCB first)

» Can be used in heart failure

» Dose: Load 0.25 mg IV every 6 hours x 4

  • Then 0.125 – 0.375 mg daily IV or PO

» Monitor dig level – therapeutic level is 0.5 – 2 ng/mL

» Adverse effects: DYSRHYTHMIAS! Heart block, bradycardia, mesenteric & myocardial ischemia

» Use cautiously in patients with hypokalemia, hypomagnesemia or hypocalcemia

» Toxicity: confusion, fatigue, ST depression, prolonged PR interval, PVCs, blurred or yellow vision, halos around objects

» If severe toxicity, can reverse with Digibind (Digoxin Immune Fab IV)

Tachyarrhythmias

Big picture – with any tachycardia, you have to think about treatable causes!

» Bleeding or hypovolemia

» ↓CO (compensatory response is to ↑HR)

» Catecholamine infusions (Epi, Dopamine, Dobutamine)

» Pain/anxiety

» Fever

Tachycardia – Narrow complex

Always ask:

» Stable vs. unstable?

» Unstable: Prepare for synchronized cardioversion!

» Stable? Narrow & regular complex?

Treatment: VAD

» Vagal maneuvers

» Diltiazem IV

» Adenosine 6 mg IV - Rapid!!!

  • (Repeat 12 mg x 2, every 1 - 2 min

Adenosine administration

» Depresses AV node conduction & SA node activity, used in SVT

» Half-life is seconds! < 10 seconds

» Dosed: 6 mg, 12 mg, 12 mg *RAPID* IVP over 1 - 2 seconds, follow by flush

  • Use IV closest to the heart

» Instruct patient prior to administration, patient may feel breathless or have transient chest pain

» Adverse effects: Transient asystole or AV block, facial flushing, hypotension, nausea (all brief)

» DO NOT use in heart blocks, WPW with wide QRS, asthma/bronchospasm

Tachycardia – Wide complex

» QRS > 0.12 sec.: consult an expert

» Amiodarone 150 mg IV over 10 min.

» Can also use Lidocaine for monomorphic wide complex tachycardia

» Monitor electrolytes
  – K^+, Mg^{++}, Ca^{++}

» AHA guidelines:

  • Adenosine 6 mg IV, may repeat dose

Antidysrhythmic Medications:

» Medications used to convert the rhythm!

» A prolonged QTc interval will be a common limiting factor with the use of anti-dysrhythmic medications!

Class	Medication	Effect	Uses
IA	Quinidine (Cardioquin)* Procainamide (Pronestyl)*	Prolongs repolarization	Atrial dys. Vent tach
IB	Lidocaine (Xylocaine)* Tocainamide (Tonocard) Mexiletin (Mexitil)	Shortens action potential duration	Ventricular Dysrhythmias
IC	Flecainamide (Tambocor) Propafenone (Rhythmol)	Blocks Na$^+$ channels	Ventricular Dysrhythmias
II	Propanolol (Inderal) Esmolol (Brevibloc)*	Decreases HR & SA node automaticity	Atrial dysrhythmias & SVT
III	Amiodarone (Cordarone)** Bretylium (Bretylol) Sotalol (Betapace)	Blocks K$^+$ channels, slows conduction	Ventricular Dysrhythmias
IV	Verapamil (Calan)* Diltiazem (Cardizem)*	Ca^{++} channel antagonist	Atrial tachycardia & atrial flutter
Other	Digoxin (Lanoxin)* Adenosine (Adenocard)*	Slows AV node conduction, depresses SA node	Afib, Aflutter & SVT

Bradyarrhythmias & Heart Blocks

» With any bradycardia, consider the cause

- Hypothermia, ischemia (think RCA!), valvular surgery (edema on the suture line), medications

» If the patient has a symptomatic bradycardia, Atropine can be attempted with caution!

- Atropine 1.0 mg IVP (per 2020 ACLS guidelines)

- Can cause tachycardia & demand ischemia

- Can also try meds with + chronotropy (Dopamine, Epi, Isuprel)

» If the patient has ongoing heart block post-op, may need a permanent pacemaker

Pacemaker Review

» Permanent or temporary

» Indications: Symptomatic bradycardia, 2nd Degree AV Block (Mobitz II), Third Degree AV Block

- Patients post aortic or mitral valve replacement are at risk of developing heart block!

» Goal: Restore A-V synchrony

- ↑CO by ↑HR!

» Modes: **Synchronous (demand)** or Asynchronous (non-demand)

- In almost all instances you want to be in Synchronous (demand) mode

- It will only pace when the patient needs it (i.e. heart rate falls below the pacemaker set rate)

- Synchronous mode avoids a pacing stimulus delivered during repolarization

  ▷ Asynchronous mode is dangerous if the patient has any underlying rhythm!!!!

  ▷ It can cause R on T leading to ventricular dysrhythmias (ventricular tachycardia, polymorphic VT or ventricular fibrillation & death

- In general, avoid asynchronous mode!

» Temporary: Demand mode should be used

» Epicardial *cardiac surgery, transcutaneous or transvenous

Epicardial Pacing Wires

» Used for emergent pacing or anytime to maintain A-V synchrony

» Stainless steel wires placed on the epicardium (outer layer)

» There is inflammation on the myocardium where the wires are placed

- Over time, will need more energy (mA)

- Usually removed POD 2 or 3

- May leave longer in valve surgery

- After about 4 – 5 days, the wires may not be effective

» Ventricular, atrial or both

- Ventricular wires placed on the right ventricle, exit skin to the left

- Atrial wires placed on the right atrium, exit skin to the right

» Always wear gloves when handling wires to prevent micro-shocks

- Often I'll touch something metal prior to handling wires

» Post wire removal, monitor for bleeding or cardiac tamponade for a few hours

- Can bleed into the pleural or epicardial space

- If orders are received to discontinue both wires & chest tubes, remove the wires 1st in case the patient bleeds

Emergent Pacing Codes:

First: Chamber paced	Second: Chamber sensed	Third: Response to sensing
A = Atrium V = Ventricle D = Dual (A & V) O = None	A = Atrium V = Ventricle D = Dual (A & V) O = None	I = Inhibited (if QRS is sensed) T = Triggered D = Inhibited & triggered O = None
TCP & TVP only able to "V" pace Epicardial – Can pace both the atria & ventricles		"I" is preferred This is Demand pacing!

Examples:

AAI mode - A: atrium is paced, A: atrium is sensed, I: pacing inhibited if the pacemaker senses intrinsic conduction

VVI mode – V: ventricle is paced, V: ventricle is sensed, I: pacing inhibited if the pacemaker senses intrinsic conduction

DDD mode – D: both atria & ventricle are paced, D: both atria & ventricle are sensed, D: pacing inhibited in both chambers if the pacemaker senses intrinsic conduction

Transcutaneous Pacing (TCP)

» External stimulation of the heart through pacing pads

» Pad placement: Anterior – posterior or anterior – lateral

Settings:

- » **Mode:** Demand (synchronous) – the only mode is VVI
  - Fixed (asynchronous) – again, AVOID!

- » **Energy:** Increase the mA (energy) until you see a pacing spike followed by a wide QRS complex
  - Set the mA above where capture was achieved (gives a safety margin)

- The wide QRS is normal because one side of the heart is being stimulated & the impulse waves across the myocardium to depolarize

- » **Rate:** There's no magic to this, if the BP is in the toilet, increase the rate!
  - Remember cardiac output = HR x SV
  - What can you manipulate? HR!
  - Assess BP to verify effective capture (BP should improve)

Other important concepts:

- » More energy required with TCP vs. transvenous or epicardial
  - For TCP, start @ 50 mA & increase until capture
  - Once capture is achieved, add an extra 10 mA to give the patient a safety margin
  - Energy requirements will vary from patient to patient

- » Not as effective as transvenous or epicardial pacing and should only be used until you can TVP!

- » Consider pain medication/ sedation as this is uncomfortable!

- » Prepare for TVP insertion if epicardial wires are not available!

Transvenous Pacing (TVP)

- » Pacing wire is inserted into the right ventricle

- » You are pacing the right side of the heart

- This naturally causes ventricular dysynchrony

- That's why we want pacers to inhibit pacing if the patient has an intrinsic rhythm

» Most wires are bipolar

- Both poles are in the heart

- The (-) pole is in contact with the myocardium

- Returns to the (+) pole

- Very small or absent pacing spike

» Less energy required vs. TCP

Initial settings:

» Always start with a new battery in the generator

» Set the **pacing mode**

- You want to be in demand mode, so the pacer can see or sense the patient's intrinsic rhythm

- We often A-V pace in Cardiac Surgery – DDD or often do AAI if in sinus brady

» Set the **pacing rate**

- ~ 60 - 80 bpm or whatever the patient needs!

» Set the **pacing output (energy)**

- Measured in milliamps (mA)

- ~ 5 mA

- Always use the lowest possible, will need more energy over time

» Set the **pacing sensitivity**

- Measured in millivolts (mV)

- ~2 mV

» If DDD pacing, set the A-V interval

- Usually ~ 170 mS

» Assess for capture – electrical (+/- pacing spike & wide QRS) & mechanical (pulse palpated)

» With any pacer setting changes, always reassess hemodynamics!

» CABG usually DDD or AAI, valve surgery usually DDD or VVI

» Secure wires

Issues with Pacing:

Failure to capture: Electrical stimulus delivered (pacing spike), but no electrical capture (wide QRS)

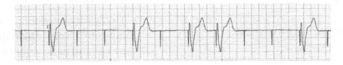

Causes:

» Improper position
  of wire or pads

» Low voltage

» Increased resistance to
  electrical stimulus

» Battery failure

» Inadequate connection

» Fibrosis of catheter tip

» Acidosis or hypoxia – may
  need higher energy setting

» Improper sensing

» Tissue inflammation

» Myocardial ischemia

Trouble-shooting:

» Check connections & battery

» Increase mA (energy)

» Try flipping the wires
  in the pacing generator
  to different poles

Failure to pace

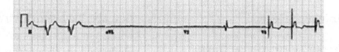

Causes:

» Battery failure

» Pad or lead dislodgement

» Improper settings

» Sensitivity is too low

Troubleshooting:

» Assess leads & connections

» Assess labs

» Change battery

» Change the generator

» Prepare for TCP

Failure to sense

Under-sensing (below): The pacemaker isn't seeing the patient's underlying rhythm

» Pacing spikes where they shouldn't be

» Need to turn down the sensitivity (mV) value, make MORE sensitive!

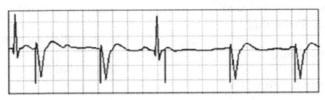

Over-sensing: Pacemaker sees events it should ignore

» Sees the P wave or the T wave & thinks it's ventricular activity

» Can also be crosstalk

» Need to increase the sensitivity (mV) value, make LESS sensitive!

Causes of sensing issues:

» Position of the lead

» *Improper sensitivity settings

» Rhythm strip above: Pacing spikes where they shouldn't be – Least sensitive

- Sensitivity setting (mV) is too high (least sensitive or asynchronous mode)

- Decrease sensitivity setting/ number (mV), making the pacemaker more sensitive!

» Can also be a sensitivity issue when pacing spikes aren't visible when they should be

- Sensitivity setting (mV) is too low (most sensitive)

- Most sensitive setting – pacer senses P & T waves & thinks they are QRS stimulus

- Increase sensitivity setting/ number (mV), making the pacemaker less sensitive!

Troubleshooting:

» Assess sensitivity threshold

Assessing Thresholds:

» Most important question to ask: Does the patient have an underlying rhythm?!

   • Can assess by slowly turning down the pacing rate

   • Can also do it by turning down the mA, but that's more risky

» Stimulation (energy) threshold

   • *Goal:* To use the least amount of energy as possible, but still capture a pacing stimulus

» Sensing threshold

   • *Goal:* Prevent competitive pacing

» Thresholds are only assessed if the patient has an underlying rhythm & is hemodynamically stable!

Stimulation (energy) Threshold:

» Increase pacing rate on generator above patients intrinsic rate

» Increase output (mA) to obtain 1:1 capture

» While watching the monitor, decrease the output (mA)

   • Note when there is no longer capture

» Increase mA until 1:1 capture resumes

   • This is the pacing threshold

   • Set mA 2 x's higher than threshold

   • Caution when mA is ≥ 10, may not increase as much for safety margin

» Return rate to previous rate setting

Sensitivity Threshold: Only if the patient is hemodynamically stable!

» Again, this is what the pacemaker "sees" or senses

» Decrease the mA to lowest setting (0.1 mA)

» Turn the pacing rate to 10 beats below the patient's intrinsic rate

» Slowly decrease the sensitivity (mV) – making it <u>more</u> sensitive (counterclockwise – smaller #)

» Watch for the flashing indicator lights

   • Green: pacing orange: sensing

» Note when the <u>sensitivity</u> indicator starts flashing with each QRS

   • This is the sensitivity threshold

   • Set the sensitivity at ½ the threshold (clockwise)

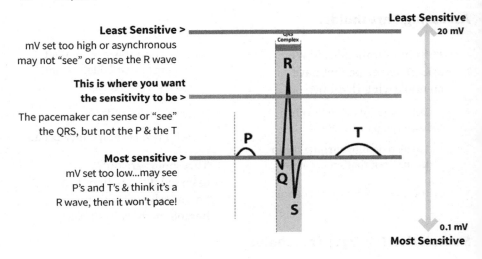

Least Sensitive >
mV set too high or asynchronous
may not "see" or sense the R wave

This is where you want
the sensitivity to be >
The pacemaker can sense or "see"
the QRS, but not the P & the T

Most sensitive >
mV set too low...may see
P's and T's & think it's a
R wave, then it won't pace!

Least Sensitive
20 mV

0.1 mV
Most Sensitive

Bottom line:

» Smaller mV value, the pacemaker sees more (most sensitive)

» Larger mV value, the pacemaker sees less (least sensitive)

Sensitivity issues:

Less or least sensitive (higher mV value)

- Pacing spikes where they shouldn't be!

- R on T & can cause arrhythmias

Too sensitive (lower mV value)

- May not pace when it needs to

- Don't see pacing spikes (or paced rhythm) when you should

You Can Do It!

Chapter 9

Pulmonary Complications

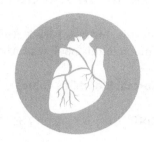

Topics covered in this chapter include:

- See Chapter 3 for Ventilator Management
- Blood gas review
- Capnography
- Acute Respiratory Distress Syndrome (ARDS)
- Transfusion-related acute lung injury (TRALI)
- Transfusion-related circulatory overload (TACO)
- Phrenic Nerve Injury
- Pneumothorax
- Air-leak syndromes (pneumomediastinum)
- Pulmonary embolism
- Pleural effusions
- Bronchospasm

Arterial Blood Gases

Know the norms & review ABG interpretation for the CSC exam. I'm not going to do much in this book with ABGs.

Normal Blood Gas Values	
pH:	7.35 - 7.45
PaO$_2$	80 - 100 (on room air)
PaCO$_2$	35 - 45
HCO$_3$	22 - 26
Base Excess	-2 to +2
SaO$_2$	95 - 100%

If the pH is < 7.35 that leans toward acidosis, > 7.45 leans toward alkalosis

If the PaCO$_2$ is < 35 that leans toward alkalosis, > 45 leans toward acidosis

If the HCO$_3$ is < 22, that leans toward acidosis, > 26 leans toward alkalosis

Post-Operative Surgical ABG derangements:

Respiratory acidosis: ↓pH/↑PaCO$_2$

» Over sedation

» Neuromuscular blockade not clearing

» Pulmonary edema

» Shivering (↑CO$_2$ production)

Metabolic acidosis: ↓pH/↓HCO$_3$

» Acute kidney injury

» ↑ lactate/hypoperfusion

» Shock

» Very elevated glucose

» Elevated electrolytes (K$^+$, Mg^{++})

Respiratory alkalosis: $\uparrow$pH/$\downarrow$PaCO$_2$

» Hyperventilation, ventilator rate too high, tidal volume too high

» Pain &/or anxiety

» Hypoxia

Metabolic alkalosis: $\uparrow$pH/$\uparrow$HCO$_3$

» Give too much bicarb

» Loop diuretics

» GI – diarrhea, vomiting, NG tube to suction

» Low electrolytes (K$^+$, Mg^{++})

Capnography - PEtCO$_2$

» Continuous with waveform

» Normal Capnography is 35 – 45 mmHg

- PEtCO$_2$ should be within 5 mm Hg of PaCO$_2$

» Is a measure of ventilation, but also a reflection of perfusion & metabolism

- If cardiac output drops, capnography values will drop

» Is the gold standard way to verify endotracheal tube placement

- Lungs vs. gut...still need a chest x-ray to determine how high or low ET tube is

» Standard of care for moderate to deep sedation

» Helpful to calculate deadspace & V/Q matching in certain conditions, like:

- Pulmonary embolus

- Pneumonia

- Over-distention of alveoli from PEEP or tidal volume

- Endotracheal tube in main stem bronchus

» As a measure of perfusion, capnography is helpful with:

- Resuscitation (CPR quality & ROSC)

- Low cardiac output states = low PEtCO$_2$

- Correlation between PEtCO$_2$ & Cardiac Output

» Other uses:

- Weaning the ventilator

- Used with PCAs/sedating agents

Pulmonary Complications

At risk:

» Smoker

» Elderly

» Pre-existing pulmonary
disease (COPD)

» Heart failure

» Obesity

» Development of pneumonia
or aspiration

Rescue:

» High flow nasal cannula (if
primarily an oxygenation issue

» CPAP – again benefits if
mostly an oxygenation issue

» BiPAP – helpful in patients with
ventilation issues (rising CO_2)

Non-Invasive Ventilation (NPPV) - BiPAP

» Continuous positive pressure

» Stabilizes airways
during exhalation

» Improves ventilation

» "Stents" alveoli open

» Used to treat:

  • COPD Exacerbation

  • CHF, pulmonary edema

  • Obstructive sleep apnea

  • Obesity hypoventilation
    syndrome

» Bi-level positive airway pressure

» CPAP that alternates
between 2 pressure levels

» Set IPAP & EPAP

» Higher mean airway pressures,
more alveolar recruitment

» Augments tidal volumes

» Typical starting point:

  • IPAP 10 cm H_2O, EPAP 5 cm H_2O

  • Inspiratory time 0.8 - 2 seconds

Acute Respiratory Distress Syndrome (ARDS)

» Inflammatory response
in the lungs

» It's rare in Cardiac Surgery
patients, but can happen

» It is not a primary disease,
but a result of:

• Cardiopulmonary bypass
  ▷ Long bypass times

• Multiple blood transfusions
(TRALI, CRALI)

• Pneumonia/aspiration

• Sepsis

What is happening in ARDS?

» INFLAMMATORY RESPONSE!

» Alveoli are infiltrated
with leukocytes

» Fibrin deposits in lungs

» Widespread endothelial
& alveolar damage

» Leaky capillaries

» Decreased compliance
(stiff lungs)

» Non-cardiogenic
pulmonary edema

Signs:

» Tachycardia

» Tachypnea, dyspnea

» Crackles or diminished
breath sounds

» Pink, watery/frothy sputum

» Progressive refractory
hypoxemia

» Worsening P/F ratio

• $(PaO_2 \div FiO_2)$

» CXR – Bilateral
pulmonary infiltrates

» Usually require mechanical
ventilation within 48°

» Hemodynamics: ↑PVR, ↑PA
pressures with normal PAOP

» What therapy will
improve the PaO_2?

• Answer: PEEP!

Diagnosis:

» Bilateral pulmonary infiltrates on CXR

» P/F Ratio: $PaO_2 \div FiO_2$

- Berlin Criteria – 2012
  ▷ < 300 – Mild ARDS
  ▷ < 200 – Moderate ARDS
  ▷ < 100 – Severe ARDS

» Predisposing conditions

» Absence of left heart failure or left atrial hypertension

» Mimics pneumonia & cardiogenic pulmonary edema

ARDS Treatment:

» Mechanical ventilation with "Lung Protective Ventilation" or "LPV"

» Lower tidal volumes; goal 6 ml/kg PBW

- Larger tidal volumes over distend & rupture distal air space (volutrauma)

- Pressure related injury (barotrauma)

- Use predicted body weight when establishing tidal volume settings

- Goal: End inspiratory plateau pressure < 30

» Allow permissive Hypercapnia

» Use of PEEP

- Think of PEEP as a stent to keep alveoli open

» When increasing PEEP, monitor for signs of decreased cardiac output!!!

- May see hypotension from increased intrathoracic chest pressure

» Use Neuromuscular blockade if dysynchrony with the ventilator

- Peripheral nerve stimulation ("Train of four") to monitor dosing

- Goal: 1 – 2 twitches out of 4 electrical stimuli

- Advantages of NM Blockade:
  ▷ Decreases barotrauma
  ▷ Decreases ventilator days
  ▷ Decreases pro-inflammatory response

Other therapies:

» Conservative fluid management

- Diuretics
- Do NOT fluid overload patients!
- Able to liberate the patient from the ventilator quicker!

» Optimize O_2 delivery

- Cardiac Output: Dobutamine or Milrinone
- PaO_2: Maximize PEEP
- Low hemoglobin: Transfuse only if necessary!

» Steroids

- No benefit from early steroids

- Some benefit days 7 – 14
- Methylprednisolone 2 – 3 mg/kg/day
- Inhibits fibrinolysis

» Prone positioning

- Newer evidence of benefit
- Must be done early, not as last ditch effort
- Should remain prone > 16 hours per day
- Risk vs. benefit with sternal wounds

» V-V ECMO to allow the lungs to rest & recover

Transfusion related acute lung injury (TRALI)

» Can happen with multiple transfusions

» Review ARDS section for signs & management

» Inflammatory process – ARDS

- Possible reaction to leukocytes

» Non-cardiogenic pulmonary edema from capillary permeability

» Does not respond to diuretics

» LPV/PEEP

Transfusion associated circulatory overload (TACO)

» CHF from too much volume from blood products!

- Basically, it's acute pulmonary edema
- Especially with rapid infusions!

- More common with FFP & platelets

» Dyspnea & crackles

» Pink, frothy sputum

» Increasing oxygen needs, desaturation

» Responsive to diuretics**

» Most patients recover quickly

Phrenic nerve injury

» Damage caused by cold cardioplegia solution

» Surgical injury or trauma to the phrenic nerve

» Can result in paralyzed diaphragm

Monitor for:

» Respiratory compromise

» Inability to wean from ventilator

» Atelectasis

» Elevated diaphragm

» Usually resolves within a few months

» Can take up to 2 years to completely resolve

Nursing Care:

» Pulmonary toileting

» Incentive spirometry

Pneumothorax

» At risk: Central lines, cannulation CPB

» Smaller pneumos, we will monitor without placing a chest tube

• All others get a chest tube!

» Absent breath sounds over the pneumo

» Trachea may deviate/shift the opposite direction

» Will have ↑ inspiratory & plateau pressures on the ventilator

Air Leak Syndromes - Pneumomediastinum

» Abnormal presence of air or another gas in the mediastinum

» Rare & usually benign

» Spontaneous <u>or</u>

» Secondary due to blunt thoracic trauma, endobronchial or esophageal procedures, head & neck surgery

Signs:

» Thoracic pain

• Usually retrosternal & pleuritic in nature

» Subcutaneous emphysema* & dyspnea

» Other symptoms may include cough, fever, dysphonia, odynophagia and dysphagia

Treatment:

» Monitor

» Rest

» Oxygen administration to dissolve air

» If symptomatic, chest tube

Pulmonary Embolus

» 70% have DVT

Signs:

» Tachycardia

» Tachypnea

» Dyspnea

» Chest pain

» Hemoptysis

» Sudden right heart failure

» Dilated right ventricle

» Cardiac Arrest

Diagnosis

» **CT Angio – detector rotated around the patient; 2-D view

- Contrast infused to view pulmonary vasculature
- 93% sensitivity / 97% specificity if clot is in one of the main arteries

Other diagnostics:

» Pulmonary angiogram

- Considered most accurate
- Performed in < 20% of patients to r/o PE because it takes too long

» Ultrasound – DVT extremities

» V/Q Scan – only diagnoses 25 – 30% of cases

- Underlying lung disease – abnormal scan

» ABG – low PaO_2

» 12 Lead ECG findings:

- Right axis deviation
- Transient right BBB
- ST depression, T wave depression in V1 – V4
- Tall peaked T waves in II, III, aVF

» D-Dimer is used only to rule out a PE

- If it's normal, it's unlikely there's a PE

Treatment:

If hemodynamically stable:

» Unfractionated Heparin (UFH)

- Weight-based dosing
- Prevent progression
- Bolus, then continuous infusion
- Goal: a PTT 60 – 100 seconds (some hospitals use anti-Xa levels)

» Warfarin

- Used with UFH
- Usually start on 1st day of Heparin therapy
- Goal: INR 2 – 3, then d/c Heparin
- Continue for 6 weeks

Can also use:

» Low Molecular Weight
   Heparin (LMWH)

» Enoxaparin 1 mg/kg Q 12 hours

* Cleared by the kidneys
  (renal adjustment)
* Simplified dosing
* No need to monitor coags
* Treat outpatient

If hemodynamic compromise:

» Hypotension / hemodynamic
   instability

» PEA Arrest

» Fibrinolytic therapy – likely
   contraindicated d/t surgery, but...

* Activase®(Alteplase) –
  0.9 mg/kg over 60 min
  not to exceed 90 mg total

* Reteplase – 10 unit IV
  bolus, repeat in 30 min
* 12% chance of major hemorrhage
* 1% ICH
* Have to weigh benefit > risk

» EKOS catheter can also
   be used (not on exam)

IVC Filters

Used if the patient has a DVT &:

» Contraindication to
   anticoagulation

» Pulmonary embolus while
   on anticoagulation

» Thrombus in right heart
   or free floating

» No DVT, but ↑ risk
   of hemorrhage

Prolonged Mechanical Ventilation

» Who's at risk?

* Prolonged metabolism &
  clearance of anesthesia

* Patients who received
  multiple transfusions

* + fluid balance

* Diaphragmatic dysfunction
  (phrenic nerve injury)

* Long CPB time

* Open chest

* Obesity

- Pre-existing impaired lung function (COPD, smokers)
- Kidney disease
- Shock
- Re-operation

» Prevent delirium

- Avoid benzodiazepines

» Assess sedation needs

- Propofol or Dexmedetomidine (Precedex) are better options if sedation is needed

» Ensure phosphate levels are adequate

- Hypophosphatemia contributes to muscle weakness

» Provide enteral nutrition ASAP!

- Protein-based
- Direct calorimetry if needed to establish CO_2 expenditure & nutritional needs

» Daily SATs with SBTs to assess readiness

Other Pulmonary Issues

Pulmonary Effusions

» Common post CPB

» If symptomatic, drain/chest tube

Bronchospasm

» Wheezing

Causes:

» Can be caused from fluid overload

» Beta blockers

» Drug interactions

» Auto-PEEP (+ pressure in distal airways)

» Hyper-inflated lungs

Treatment:

» Beta$_2$ agonist (Albuterol)

» Steroids

» Magnesium (relaxes airways)

» Lower tidal volume

» If ventilated, allow longer time in exhalation if air trapping

» If laryngospasm, nebulized racemic epinephrine is usually help

You Can Do It!

Chapter 10

All other systems

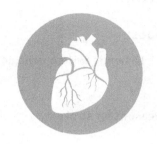

Topics covered in this chapter include:

- Stroke
- Carotid Stenosis/Endartectomy
- Acute kidney injury (ATN, azotemia)
- Electrolyte imbalances
- Delirium
- Ischemic bowel

Stroke

Types:

» Ischemic & Hemorrhagic

» Stroke incidence is about 3% post cardiac surgery

Reasons for stroke:

» Blood clots

» Atrial fibrillation

- Left atrial or left ventricular thrombus

» Atherosclerotic plaque embolism

» Air embolism from CPB

» Decreased perfusion during surgery

» Cerebral edema

» Conversion of embolic to hemorrhagic

AHA Stroke Guidelines

» 1 hour goals:

- Complete NIH Stroke Scale Assessment

- Treatment with fibrinolytic therapy isn't going to be possible in most cases since they are post-surgical

- Mechanical Thrombectomy should be considered!

- Anticoagulation with heparin

NIH Stroke Scale assesses:

» LOC

» Eye deviation (CN III, VI, VIII)

» Visual field loss (hemianopia)

» Facial palsy

» Motor arms (drift)

» Motor legs

» Limb ataxia

» Sensory

» Language

» Dysarthria

» Extinction & inattention

Diagnostics

» CT scan <u>without</u> contrast

 • R/O hemorrhage

 • Should be interpreted within 45 min

 • Might see hypodensity in ischemic area

» CT perfusion or MRI perfusion

» Measures infarct core or penumbra

» Non-invasive intra-cranial vascular study if plan to do intra-arterial fibrinolysis or mechanical thrombectomy

Endovascular therapies for Ischemic Stroke

» Newer evidence to combine rtPA with endovascular procedures

» May be reasonable in patients with a contraindication to IV fibrinolysis (i.e. Surgical patients)

» Intra-arterial rtPA may also be considered

Stroke care components

» Cardiac monitoring

 • Atrial fibrillation & cardiac arrhythmias

» Restart anti-hypertensives after 24 hours

» Airway support

 • Ventilatory assistance if needed

 • Apply O_2 only if needed, if O_2 sats are < 94%

 • Aspiration risk

» Avoid fever!!! (temp > 38°C)

 • Antipyretic therapy

» Treat hypovolemia

» Treat hypoglycemia (< 70 mg/dL)

 • Goal: normoglycemia

 • BS 140 – 180 mg/dL (or tighter)

 • Worse outcomes if hyperglycemic or hypoglycemic

» DVT prophylaxis

 • SCDs or prophylactic anticoagulation

 • Early mobilization

» NPO until swallow evaluation

- Nurse-driven swallow screen

- If unable to take solids, consider placing a feeding tube

- If > 2 weeks, consider PEG

» Avoid in-dwelling urinary catheters

- High risk of UTIs specifically in the neuro population

Nursing considerations for stroke care:

» Frequent neuro checks

- Monitor for signs of increased ICP

- Placement of a Ventriculostomy drain if develop hydrocephalus

- Prophylactic anti-convulsants are not recommended

» Corticosteroids are not routinely recommended

» Monitor for seizures

» Monitor for bleeding with anticoagulation

Carotid Stenosis

» Often patients who need Cardiac Surgery have some degree of Carotid Stenosis

» Evaluated pre-op on many patients

» If the carotid is not treated pre-op, may need higher BP post-op for perfusion

Clinical presentation:

» TIAs, visual Δ's

» Memory loss

» Vertigo, syncope

» Bruit or thrill

Treatment:

» Antiplatelet aggregation (ASA, Plavix)

» BP control

- Specific patient targets should be established

- Do not want to drop too much

» Balloon angioplasty (not done as much)

Carotid Endarterectomy

» Post-op: Monitor for bleeding/hematoma

» Close airway monitoring (location of incision)

» Neuro assessment

» Cranial nerve assessment:

- VII: Smile
- IX/X: Swallow, gag, speech
- XI: Shrug shoulders
- XII: Stick out tongue

Renal Dysfunction - Acute Kidney Injury (AKI)

» a.k.a. Acute renal failure (ARF)

» Abrupt decline in glomerular filtration rate (GFR)

» Results in retention of metabolic waste

- Protein catabolism (azotemia)
- Electrolyte & acid-base imbalance (retention of potassium, magnesium & phosphate, acidosis)
- Fluid overload

Causes of AKI:

» Low perfusion, medications

» Reversible if prompt treatment is received

Labs to assess in AKI:

» BUN & creatinine

- Up to 12 hour lag time in elevation. Not an early indicator!

» BUN/Creatinine ratio, normal ratio is 10:1 to 15:1

» Glomerular Filtration Rate (estimated by creatinine clearance)

- Normal creatinine clearance is about 80 – 120 ml/min

» Urinalysis:

- Casts - Presence is a sign of tubular cell death
- Electrolytes (specifically Na^+)
- Albumin
- Glucose
- Protein

Prerenal AKI

» Results from hypoperfusion

» Kidney structure & function is preserved

» Causes: Sepsis, heart failure, trauma, severe hypovolemia

» BUN/Creatinine ratio > 20:1 (BUN elevates, creatinine may start to elevate)

» Oliguria

» Urine Na^+ < 20 mEq/L (kidneys hold on to Na^+ & H_2O)

» Urine osmo & urine specific gravity ↑ due to concentration

» HIGH RISK for progressing to ATN!

» Treatment: Treat cause, improve perfusion!

Acute Tubular Necrosis (ATN)

» May also be referred to "intrarenal" kidney injury

» Injury occurs at the nephron; there is structural damage!

» Causes: Hypotension, glomerulonephritis, diabetes, rhabdomyolysis, nephrotoxic medications, shock states

» BUN/Creatinine ratio 10:1
  • Both BUN & creatinine are elevated

» BUN > 25 mg/dL, creatinine > 1.2 mg/dL

» Often requires renal replacement therapy (RRT)

Treatment:

» Depends on cause, assess if dialysis is indicated

» Prevent acidosis, electrolyte imbalance & uremia!

» Stop nephrotoxic medications!

Indications for Dialysis

Easy acronym to remember reasons:

A: Acid/base imbalance

E: Electrolyte imbalance (hyperkalemia, hypermagnesemia, hyperphosphatemia)

I: Intoxications (ODs/toxins)

O: Overload (fluid)

U: Uremic symptoms

Laboratory findings in ATN in need of RRT:

» BUN > 35

» Creatinine > 4 or, creatinine climbing ≥ 1 point/day

» Uncompensated metabolic acidosis

» Anemia

» Electrolyte imbalances
  • Increased potassium (> 6.5), magnesium, phosphate
  • Decreased calcium, bicarb
  • Abnormal urine electrolytes

Uremic Syndrome symptoms (when the BUN is elevated)

» Neurologic: Lethargy, fatigue, seizures, coma

» Cardiovascular: ECG changes (d/t hyperkalemia),signs of fluid overload; tachycardia, S3 heart sound, hypo/hypertension

» Hematologic: Anemia

» Pulmonary: Crackles, pulmonary edema, SOB, effusions, pleuritis from uremia

» Gastrointestinal: Decreased appetite, nausea & vomiting, ascites & fluid overload

General Treatment Goals for AKI

» Hemodynamic stability

» Improve renal perfusion

» Correct chemistry abnormalities
(electrolytes, BUN, creatinine)

» Monitor electrolyte imbalances

- During therapy

- After therapy

» Adequate hydration

- Careful use of diuretics

- Accurate, meticulous
daily weights

» Aggressive dialysis

» Monitor drug levels for toxicity

» Monitor coags

» Alter medication schedules
around dialysis if needed

» Modify medication dosing
– identify meds cleared
through kidneys

» Minimize exposure to
nephrotoxic medications

» Prevent infection

» Maintain nutritional state

Contrast induced nephropathy (CIN)

Highest risk patients:

» Diabetics, HTN, heart failure

» Pre-existing renal insufficiency

» Dehydrated

» Concurrent use of nephrotoxic
medications (i.e. NSAIDS,
ACE Inhibitors)

» High volume of IV contrast

» 10% of all patients who
receive IV contrast dye
develop CIN – yikes!

» ***HYDRATION!!! is the
key to prevention***

- A little rhyme to remember:
The solution to pollution
(contrast dye) is dilution!!!!

- Hydrate to protect the kidneys!!!

» Sodium bicarbonate infusion
– 1 hour before & 6 hours after
exposure to contrast dye

- Not much evidence
to support this

» N-Acetylcysteine (Mucomyst) for prevention (stinky!)

- 600 mg PO day before & day of contrast exposure (total of 4 doses)

- Thought to prevent toxicity to renal tubules

- Not much evidence to support this

Dialysis

Hemodialysis Complications

» Hypotension

» Dysrhythmias (d/t electrolyte shifts)

» Angina

» Fever from pyrogenic reaction

» Coagulopathy, thrombocytopenia

» Disequilibrium Syndrome (post-treatment cerebral edema)

» Air embolism

Air Embolism

Venous signs:

» Shortness of breath

» Chest pain

» Acute right heart failure (if obstructs blood flow from right heart to the lungs)

» Looks like a Pulmonary Embolism!

Treatment:

» Lay on left side, trendelenburg position

» Oxygenate with with 100% FiO_2

- Accelerates the removal of nitrogen in the air embolism

Arterial signs:

- » Change in LOC (looks like a stroke!)

- » Decreased arterial flow and perfusion (looks like an occluded artery)

- It only takes 2 ml of air to be fatal in an artery

- Only 0.5 ml air to be fatal in a coronary artery

- » Oxygenate with 100% FiO_2

Continuous Renal Replacement Therapy (CRRT)

- » Slow continuous fluid removal

- » Used in patients who are hemodynamically unstable

- » Must have sufficient mean arterial pressure (MAP) or AV gradient to run CRRT

- AV Gradient is calculated by using the MAP – CVP

- > 60 mm Hg is desired

- » If the AV gradient is too low, vasopressors may be needed to increase the blood pressure

- » Indications: fluid removal refractory to diuretics

Complications:

- » Hypotension

- » Bleeding (anticoagulation)

- » Hypothermia – can use a warmer

- » Filter/circuit clotting

- » Membrane rupture (blood in effluent bag)

- Immediately stop treatment & disconnect!

Electrolyte Imbalances

Sodium

- » Normal 135 – 145 mEq/L

- » Sodium is important for fluid balance in the body

- » Often follow serum osmolality if there are fluid balance concerns

Hypernatremia Na⁺ > 145 mEq/L

Causes:

» Dehydration, water loss

» Excess administration of NaCl, hypertonic saline or $NaHCO_3$

» Hypertonic enteral feedings

» Diabetes insipidus

Symptoms:

» Thirst, tachycardia, hypotension, restless, irritable, lethargy, muscle weakness, flushed skin, oliguria (with dehydration)

» May also see increased hematocrit (hemo-concentrated)

» Increased Chloride

• Often > 106 mEq/L

» Increased serum osmolality

» Increased urine specific gravity due to concentrated urine in dehydration

• Often > 1.025

» Decreased urine Na⁺

Treatment:

» Fluid hydration

» Free H_2O

» Hypotonic IV solution (.45 saline)

» Diuretics (to remove sodium) – of appropriate for cause

Hyponatremia – Na⁺ < 132 mEq/L

Causes:

» Excess H_2O or Na⁺ depletion

» Water retention

» NG tube suction

» SIADH – dilutional hyponatremia

» Diarrhea

» Intestinal surgery

» DKA

» Heart, liver or renal failure

Symptoms:

» Neuro changes, headache, confusion, cerebral edema, coma, death

» Anxiety, weakness, seizures, hypotension, tachycardia, shock

» Abdominal cramping, nausea, weight gain

» Shortness of breath, crackles

» Low hemoglobin (dilutional effect)

Treatment:

» Slow Na^+ correction!!!!

  • No more than 8 – 12 mEq/day

» Na^+ Phosphate 1 – 2 mmol/ hour over 3 – 4 hours

» Hypertonic saline

» Na^+ tabs

» If water excess, diuresis

Potassium

» Normal K^+ levels: 3.5 – 5.0 mEq/L

» 90% intracellular, 10% in serum

» Na^+/K^+ pump – maintains normal cell volume and electroneutrality of the cell membrane

Functions of K^+:

» Transmission of nerve impulses

» Intracellular osmolality

» Enzymatic reactions

» Acid-base balance

» Myocardial, skeletal & smooth muscle contractility

Potassium Regulation

» Kidneys – Primary excretory source

  • So efficient rarely have hyper states in normal renal function

  • In the presence of aldosterone, K is excreted by the renal tubules

» Intestines – excrete K^+

Hypokalemia: < 3.5 mEq/L

Causes:

» Diuresis - increased urinary loss

» Magnesium depletion

» Insulin

» GI: Vomiting, NGT suctioning (aggravated by metabolic alkalosis)

» Diarrhea, fistula, ileostomy

» Hyperaldosterone states, thiazide diuretics, amphotericin, gentamycin

» Inadequate intake

» Anorexia, ETOH

Symptoms:

» Clinical presentation – develop symptoms when K^+ < 3.2 mEq/L

» Cardiovascular irritability

- Ventricular irritability (PVCs) < 2.8

- PACs

» Ventricular fibrillation

» Depressed ST segment

» Development of a u-wave

» Prolonged QT interval

» Potentiates Digoxin activity

» Muscle cramping, weakness

» Intracellular shift causing Alka-*LO*-sis

- 0.1 unit ↑ in pH, causes ↓ K^+ by 0.4 mEq/L

Treatment:

» Replace K^+

» Oral supplements or increased dietary intake when possible

» IV - Standard dose 10 - 20 mEq over 1 – 2 hours

- Central line administration preferred

» Eliminate or treat conditions that promote K^+ shifts (i.e. alkalosis)

» Ensure adequate renal function

» *ALWAYS think about Magnesium replacement if appropriate!

Hyperkalemia K⁺ > 5.5 mEq

Causes:

» Renal failure (~75% of all cases)

- Inability of renal tubules to excrete K⁺

» Acidosis

» Decreased cardiac output

» Cardioplegia solution

» Hemolysis of blood from CPB

» K⁺ sparing diuretics

Symptoms:

» Nausea & vomiting

» Diarrhea

» Tingling skin

» Numbness in hands & feet

» Flaccid paralysis

» Apathy, confusion

Cardiac symptoms:

» Tall tented/peaked symmetrical T waves (K⁺ > 6.5)

» Widened QRS, prolonged PR, widened P wave (K⁺ > 8.0)

» Decreased automaticity (K⁺ 9.0 - 11.0)

» P waves disappear

» QRS merges with T to form sine wave

» Bradycardia

- Challenging to pace, will need more energy

» Asystole or ventricular fibrillation

» Decreased strength of cardiac contraction

Treatment: Emergency (move/shift potassium)

» Regular Insulin IV

- Dextrose if normal or low glucose to prevent hypoglycemia

» NaHCO₃ – not as efficient as insulin

- Use only if acidosis is present

» Nebulized albuterol

- Onset ~15 min., duration about 15 – 90 min.

» Calcium chloride or gluconate (cardiac protectant; no effect on K^+ levels)

Removal of potassium:

» Dialysis *

» Loop diuretics (functioning kidneys)

» Sodium polystyrene sulfonate (Kayexalate)

- Dose 15 grams 1 - 4 doses/day (PO, FT, PR)
- 24 hours to correct
- Shouldn't be used for emergent treatment

Magnesium

» Normal level 1.5 – 2.5 mEq/L

» Generally in cardiac patients, we keep the Mg^{++} level on the higher/normal side

Functions:

» Neuromuscular transmission

» Cardiac contraction

Hypomagnesemia < 1.4 mEq/L

Causes:

» Diuretics: blocks Na^+ reabsorption

» Increased excretion

» Hypokalemia

- Mg^{++} inhibits the release of K^+ & ↑ K^+ losses
- If K^+ is low, replace the Mg^{++} 1st!

» NG suctioning, diarrhea, fistulas

» Osmotic diuresis

» Antibiotics

» Decreased intake

» Chronic alcoholism

» Malabsorption

Symptoms:

» CV: Tachycardia, depressed ST segment, ↓CO

» Atrial & ventricular arrhythmias

- PACs & PVCs

» Torsades de Pointes! Caused by prolonged QT!

- Polymorphic ventricular tachycardia

» Hypotension

» Coronary artery spasm

» Neuromuscular

- Twitching, paresthesia, cramps, muscle tremors

- + Chvostek & Trousseau's signs

» CNS: mentation changes, seizures

» Hypokalemia

Treatment:

» IV 1 - 2 grams $MgSO_4$ over 60 minutes

- Emergency give over 1 - 2 minutes (Torsades)

- Monitor BP & airway when administering magnesium!

- Can get hypotensive & flushed with Mg^{++}

» Assess renal function

» Increase Mg^{++} intake

» Increased risk for digoxin toxicity

» Dietary: diet or PO supplementation

- Add to IV or TPN

» Monitor neurological status

» Monitor K^+ and Ca^{++}

» Follow serial magnesium levels

Hypermagnesemia > 2.5 mEq/L

Causes:

» Decreased excretion from renal failure is the most common

» Can also see in acidosis, DKA

Symptoms:

» 3 - 5 mEq/L Peripheral dilation, facial flushing, hypotension

» 4 - 7 mEq/L Drowsiness, lethargy

» When Mg^{++} is elevated, patients get the "Mag Drag"! (Lethargy, drowsy)

Treatment:

» Increase excretion of Mg^{++} by using fluids & diuretics

» If impaired renal function - Dialysis

Hypocalcemia – Ca++ < 8.5

» Follow **ionized** (active) Ca^{++}

• Normal: 1.1 – 1.35 mmol/L

Causes:

» Diarrhea

» Diuretics

» Malabsorption

» Chronic renal failure

» Alkalosis; Ca^{++} bound to albumin & is inactive

» Phosphate & calcium have an inverse relationship to each other!

Symptoms:

» CV: Prolonged QTc, ↓BP, ↓CO, ventricular ectopy, ventricular fibrillation

» Neuromuscular: Tingling, spasms, tetany, seizures

 • Twitching, paresthesia, cramps, muscle tremors

 • + Chvostek & Trousseau's signs

» Respiratory: Bronchospasm; labored shallow breathing

» Gastrointestinal: smooth muscle hyperactivity

» Bleeding; Ca^{++} needed to clot

 • Ca^{++} is Factor IV

» Safety: confusion & seizures

» Muscle cramps can precede tetany

Treatment:

» Administer calcium
chloride or gluconate

Hypophosphatemia < 2.5 mg/dL

» Necessary for cellular energy

» Tissue catabolism: increase
use in tissue repair

» Low levels = muscle weakness!

Causes:

» Decreased intake

» ETOH

» Hypothermia

» Increased elimination

» Vomiting and diarrhea

» Pre-op use of phosphate
binding antacids

» Increased urinary
losses: osmotic diuresis,
thiazide diuretics

» Increased utilization or
Intracellular shifts

» Alkalosis (respiratory)

» Refeeding syndrome
  • See when patient has been
    NPO & nutrition is restarted

Symptoms: (secondary to decreases in ATP & 2,3 DPG)

Acute:

» ↓BP, CO & SV

» Confusion, seizures, coma

» Chest pain due to poor
oxygenation of the myocardium

» Numbness and tingling of the
fingers, circumoral region

» Incoordination

» Speech difficulty

» Weakness of respiratory muscle
  • May prolong mechanical
    ventilation
  • ↓ contraction of the diaphragm

Chronic:

» Memory loss, lethargy

» Bone pain

» Hypomagnesemia

Treatment:

» Identification and
elimination of the cause

» Increase dietary intake
of phosphate

» Oral phosphate supplements

• K^+ or Na^+ phosphate capsules

» IV: potassium phosphate
or sodium phosphate

Hyperphosphatemia > 4.5 mg/dL

Causes:

» Increased intake from
phosphate containing antacids

» Decreased excretion
- renal failure

» Transcellular shifts

» Respiratory acidosis,
intracellular release

» Cell lysis of RBC, skeletal
muscle or tumor cells

Symptoms:

» Rebound hypocalcemia

» phosphate binds with
free calcium and ionized
serum calcium falls

» Ectopic disposition of $Ca\text{-}PO_4$

» Anorexia, nausea, vomiting

» Muscle weakness,
hyperreflexia, tetany

» Tachycardia

» $\uparrow PO_4 = \downarrow Ca^{++}$

Treatment:

» Identification and elimination of cause

» Use of aluminum, magnesium or calcium gels or antacids: binds phosphorus in the gut

» Avoid meats, fish, poultry, milk, whole grains, seeds, nuts, eggs, dried beans

» Dialysis therapy

» Acetazolamide stimulated urinary PO_4 excretion

Delirium

» Acute brain dysfunction

» Key characteristics:
  • Inattention
  • Confusion

• Disorganized thinking

• Can wax & wane

• Hyperactive & hypoactive (more common)

Who is at risk?

» Hospitalized patients

» Elderly

» Post CPB patients!!!!

» Stroke, CNS issues

» Sepsis

» Sleep deprived

» Electrolyte imbalances

» Dehydration

» Memory impaired

Monitoring for delirium

» Confusion Assessment Method (CAM) – ICU Assessment

» Most validated tool & widely used

» Assess for fluctuation in neuro status from baseline

» Assess RASS (or sedation level)

PADIS Guidelines – Updated in 2018

» Guidelines to give direction on delirium prevention & treatment

Pain

» Treat pain first!!!

» Multi-modal approach to pain management

» Use a behavioral pain assessment scale

» Ask the right questions

» Do not use sedatives to treat pain

» Pre-emptive pain plan for:
  • Treatments
  • Mobility – Dressing change

Agitation

» Minimize sedation

» Avoid benzodiazepines
  • Unless ETOH withdrawal

» Consider non-benzodiazepines for sedation
  • Propofol
  • Dexmetomidine (Precedex)

» Don't overuse sedation; "light" sedation

  • RASS -1 to 0 should be the goal

» Avoid "deep" sedation unless absolutely clinically warranted

» Daily interruption in sedation (wake patient up)

» Determine sedation goal

» Consider non-pharmacologic interventions

Delirium

» Monitor for it!!!

» Prevent it!!!

» Identify who is at risk

» If the patient develops delirium:
  • Identify reversible causes
  • Avoid benzodiazepines
  • Dexmetomidine (Precedex) associated with lower delirium risk vs. benzo

» Review their medication
list – eliminate any
meds not necessary

» Pharmacist consult

Immobility

Sleep Disturbances

General prevention considerations:

» Glasses & hearing aids
on the patient!

» Day/night orientation

» Mobilize the patient
ASAP post-op!!!

» Method of communicating
if barrier

» Reorientation frequently

» Board in room with place & date

» Clock in view

» Noise control

» Promote sleep

» Cluster care activities

Bowel Ischemia

» Associated with
decreased C.O. or BP

• At risk: patients with heart
failure, low C.O. state

• Ischemia is secondary to
overall low perfusion state

Intestinal Ischemia/Infarction Diagnosis:

» History & clinical presentation

» Rule out other causes

» CT scan – assess for free
air (perforation)

» Radiographic Angiography

» Assess for embolus or thrombus

» Surgery

• Assess for ischemic or infarcted
bowel (more difficult)

Labs:

» Nonspecific

» Leukocytosis

» Elevated lactate (sign of tissue hypoxia)

» Elevated LDH, amylase

» ABG (metabolic acidosis)

Treatment:

» Improve cardiac output!

» Adequate resuscitation

» Vasodilator therapy to dilate the mesenteric artery

» Surgery - Resect infarcted bowel

» Follow serial lactate levels as a marker of perfusion

You Can Do It!

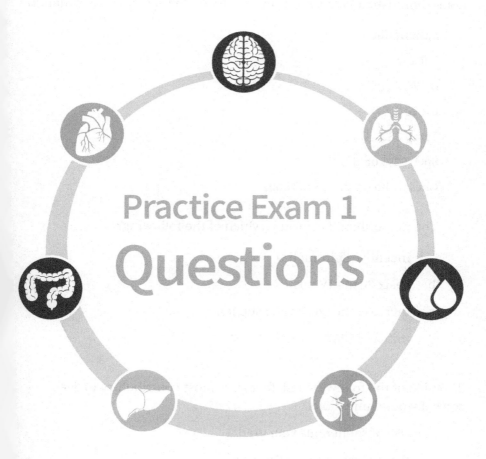

Practice Exam 1
Questions

Practice Exam 1

1. The nurse is assessing a patient 12-hours post cardiac surgery and notes diminished lung sounds in the bilateral bases upon auscultation.

Patient data:

HR 102

BP 98/52 (67)

RR 22

Temp 38.2° C

SpO_2 92% on 5 L NC

Chest tube output 15 ml/hour

The nurse should prioritize which of the following?

a. Incentive spirometry

b. Lasix 20 mg IV push

c. Increase the chest tube suction

d. Initiate BiPAP

2. Which of the following risk factors is most contributory to deep sternal wound infections?

a. Use of saphenous vein graft

b. Peripheral Vascular Disease

c. Obesity

d. Neuropathy

3. A 74-year-old male receives a left ventricular assist device (LVAD) for worsening end stage heart failure. Upon return to the Cardiothoracic Intensive Care Unit (CTICU) post device implantation, the nurse should assess for which of the following complications immediately post-operative?

    a.   Acquired von Willebrand Syndrome

    b.   Infection

    c.   Bleeding

    d.   GI obstruction

4. After undergoing an uncomplicated transcatheter aortic valve replacement (TAVR), the nurse understands the most common dysrhythmia to monitor for is:

    a.   Ventricular fibrillation

    b.   Junctional rhythm

    c.   Atrial fibrillation

    d.   Complete heart block

5. A 43-year-old female patient with von Willebrand's Type I disease is 5 hours postoperative from an aortic valve replacement. She is experiencing continued bleeding via her mediastinal chest tubes and is hypotensive. Her coagulation panel has been corrected and she received Factor VIII. The RN should anticipate the addition of which medication?

    a.   Desmopressin

    b.   Amicar

    c.   Cryoprecipitate

    d.   Norepinephrine

6. Two hours after open heart surgery for triple vessel disease, a patient is suspected of developing cardiogenic shock. Which of the following hemodynamic profiles is consistent with cardiogenic shock from left ventricular pump failure?

    a.   Decreased cardiac index, decreased SVR, decreased PAOP, decreased CVP

    b.   Decreased cardiac index, increased SVR, increased PAOP, increased CVP

    c.   Decreased cardiac index, decreased SVR, increased PAOP, decreased CVP

    d.   Decreased cardiac index, increased SVR, increased PAOP, decreased CVP

7. You are caring for a 67-year-old male s/p aortic valve replacement (AVR) and redo CABG. He has had mediastinal bleeding > 150 ml/hour for the past 3 hours. During the last hour, there was no chest tube drainage. Which of the following signs would raise concern for cardiac tamponade?

    a.   Increased filling pressures, decreased cardiac output, wide pulse pressure

    b.   Decreased filling pressures, decreased cardiac output, hypotension

    c.   Decreased filling pressures, decreased pulmonary occlusion pressure (PAOP), wide pulse pressure

    d.   Increased filling pressures, decreased cardiac output, narrow pulse pressure

8. A patient who is one hour post cardiac surgery has a sudden rhythm change during endotracheal suctioning. The following rhythm is visualized on the bedside monitor:

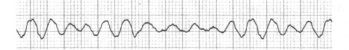

The patient is immediately defibrillated with 3 stacked shocks per CALS protocol and chest compressions are started. A femoral pulse is palpable with compressions. Capnography monitoring is initiated and shows a PetCO$_2$ of 8 mm Hg. The appropriate action by the code leader is:

    a. Increase the frequency of assisted ventilations via bag valve mask.

    b. Halt compressions and assess for return of spontaneous circulation (ROSC).

    c. Assess the quality of compressions.

    d. Apply a pulse oximeter to assess ventilation.

9. Why is an aortic valve replacement the preferred method over a repair with diseased aortic valves?

    a. Less post-operative complications due to less time spent in the OR.

    b. Better ability for the heart to re-modulate and recovery is more stable.

    c. Leaflet fibrosis and retraction occurs with repair, leading to aortic regurgitation.

    d. Better life expectancy with the increased durability of a replacement.

10. During the bedside handoff, the nurse caring for a new post-operative CABG patient is told that bilateral internal mammary arteries were used as grafts. The right internal mammary (RIMA) bypassed the right coronary artery (RCA) and the left internal mammary (LIMA) bypassed the LAD. Because both mammary arteries were used as bypass grafts, what will be a priority in nursing care?

    a. Aggressive pulmonary toileting

    b. Bilateral upper extremity neurovascular checks

    c. Hourly neurological checks

    d. Meticulous sternal incision care

11. A 69-year-old female patient is 6 hours post-operative from a mitral valve repair. The patient has been experiencing some bleeding and remains intubated on the ventilator. Her initial hemoglobin was 6.1 g/dL with a hematocrit of 18%. The surgeon ordered 3 units of PRBCs for the low blood count.

During the administration of the 3rd unit of PRBCs, the patient becomes hypertensive with a blood pressure of 190/100 mm Hg. The patient is not responsive to vasodilator therapy. The SpO_2 is now reading 88%, despite increasing the FiO_2 to 100% on the ventilator. The nurse should anticipate which of the following therapies?

   a.   Furosemide (Lasix) 40 mg IVP

   b.   An additional unit of PRBCs

   c.   Addition of a second vasodilator

   d.   Increase the PEEP on the ventilator

12. Which of the following is an advantage of having an off-pump Coronary Artery Bypass Graft (CABG) surgery?

   a.   Reduced risk of bleeding

   b.   Increased graft patency

   c.   Reduced risk for neurological complications

   d.   Reduced risk for revascularization

13. The nurse is caring for a patient one hour post single vessel CABG. The patient is intubated with a central venous catheter (CVC) in place. On assessment, peripheral pulses are palpable, but weak with capillary refill time < 3 seconds.

Patient data:

HR 120

BP 80/44 (56)

T 36.5° C

CVP 2 mm Hg

HCT 32%, Hgb 10.5

Chest tube output: 100 ml total

The nurse should anticipate which of the following orders from the provider?

    a.   Two units packed red blood cells transfused stat.

    b.   One liter of lactated ringers IV bolus.

    c.   A chest radiograph to verify chest tube placement.

    d.   Norepinephrine to maintain the systolic BP > 95 mm Hg.

14. A patient is being evaluated for a CABG following an acute anteroseptal myocardial infarction four days prior. On admission, the patient is stable and has a Pulmonary Artery catheter (PAC) in place. The nurse reassesses the patient four hours later and notices a new holosystolic murmur and an abrupt rise in the pulmonary artery pressures. What is the mostly likely explanation for these acute findings?

    a.   Acute mitral valve prolapse

    b.   Acute ventricular septal rupture

    c.   Left ventricular free wall rupture

    d.   Pseudoaneurysm of the left ventricle

15. A 43-year-old female patient has recently returned from the OR after a 2 vessel CABG with bypasses to the LAD and RCA. The nurse is sending routine post-op labs. Which lab findings should the nurse anticipate?

    a.   Hypocalcemia, hypokalemia, hypomagnesemia, hypophosphatemia

    b.   Hypocalcemia, hyperkalemia, hypomagnesemia, hyperphosphatemia

    c.   Hypercalcemia, hyperkalemia, hypermagnesemia, hypophosphatemia

    d.   Hypercalcemia, hypokalemia, hypomagnesemia, hyperphosphatemia

16. Your unit has a goal of early extubation, ideally within 6 hours of CABG surgery. To achieve successful early extubation, patients must be weaned based on clinical condition, not based on time or unit routines. Which of the following criteria would exclude your patient from early extubation?

    a.   Minimal chest tube output

    b.   Patient is anxious, writing notes

    c.   Increasing the Epinephrine infusion for hypotension

    d.   Bradycardia with a heart rate of 48 requiring pacing on standby

17. A patient is 3 hours post cardiac surgery. A pulmonary artery catheter is in place and 2 mediastinal chest tubes are patent to -20 cm suction. The chest tube output suddenly increases to 300 ml per hour. Which of the following hemodynamic profiles would the nurse anticipate in response to hypovolemia from bleeding?

    a.   CI 2.2 L/min/m², CVP 9 mm Hg, PAOP 14 mm Hg, HR 98

    b.   CI 1.9 L/min/m², CVP 2 mm Hg, PAOP 6 mm Hg, HR 120

    c.   CI 1.8 L/min/m², CVP 12 mm Hg, PAOP 18 mm Hg, HR 70

    d.   CI 2.0 L/min/m², CVP 15 mm Hg, PAOP 20 mm Hg, HR 145

18. A 35-year-old male is 3 hours post-op from a 3 vessel CABG with full median sternotomy and is mechanically ventilated. His medical history is significant for hyperlipidemia, hypertension and Type 1 Diabetes Mellitus. The nurse notices as the patient is starting to wake, his heart rate is 112 and arterial blood pressure is 162/70 mm Hg. What is the most appropriate initial action to treat the hypertension?

    a.   Assess and treat pain

    b.   Assess closed drainage unit for increases in chest tube drainage

    c.   Prepare to initiate Nitroglycerin infusion at 10 mcg/min and titrate to keep the MAP > 65 mm Hg

    d.   Review the home medication list and notify the provider to restart the home antihypertensive medications

19. Post-operatively, a 39-year-old female patient develops atrial fibrillation with a rapid ventricular response and rate in the 180s with symptomatic hypotension and chest pain. The RN should anticipate which of the following interventions?

    a.   Synchronized Cardioversion

    b.   Amiodarone infusion

    c.   Diltiazem infusion

    d.   Digoxin IVP

20. A postoperative CABG patient is being transvenous paced at 90 bpm in VVI mode. The nurse assesses skin integrity and turns the patient to their right side. While turned to the right, the patient complains of chest pain and shortness of breath. The nurse looks at the monitor to find the patient is no longer paced, with a brady rhythm at 36 bpm.

    What is the first immediate action the nurse should take?

    a.   Return the patient to their original position

    b.   Activate a Code Blue

    c.   Increase the pacemaker mA (energy) setting

    d.   Continue to assess the skin while reassuring the anxious patient

21. Which of the following is the most common adverse outcome following coronary artery bypass graft surgery (CABG)?

    a.   Renal failure

    b.   Mediastinitis

    c.   Anemia

    d.   Vein graft failure

22. Upon receiving a patient post 2-vessel CABG with an aortic valve replacement, the Anesthesiologist reports the patient was on cardiopulmonary bypass for more than 3 hours. The patient is hypotensive despite receiving autologous blood and 500 ml of 5% albumin. The Epinephrine infusion dose was increased. The cardiac index is 2.9 L/min/m^2, CVP 6 mm Hg, PAOP 10 mm Hg, SVR 450 dynes/sec/cm^{-5}. You are concerned the patient may be experiencing Vasoplegic shock. Considering this, which of the following medications would be most beneficial?

    a. Dopamine

    b. Dobutamine

    c. Vasopressin

    d. Milrinone

23. A diabetic patient with known left ventricular dysfunction is admitted following a myocardial infarction. She was found to have 3-vessel coronary disease and anemia. While awaiting coronary artery bypass graft (CABG), the provider orders a unit of packed red blood cells. Hours after the blood was transfused, the nurse notices the patient is hypertensive and short of breath without fever, chills, or hives on exam. After notifying the provider, the nurse would anticipate which of the following?

    a. Place the patient in reverse Trendelenburg position to treat the low blood pressure.

    b. Administer diuretics for volume overload due to a history of heart failure with reduced ejection fraction.

    c. Administer Benadryl for a potential blood transfusion reaction.

    d. Administer a cardiac inotrope due to history of left ventricular dysfunction.

24. An 88-year old female is being admitted from the Operating Room after a Thoracic Endovascular Aortic Repair (TEVAR). Which interventions should the nurse prioritize to minimize the risk of developing delirium?

    a. Place a vest restraint for the night

    b. Administer a PRN sleep aid

    c. Remove unnecessary invasive devices

    d. Maintain minimal room lightening and quiet during the day

25. An intra-aortic balloon pump (IABP) would be indicated for which of the following patients?

    a. Papillary Muscle Rupture

    b. Aortic Insufficiency

    c. Thoracic Aneurysm

    d. Tricuspid Stenosis

26. An 80-year-old female is to undergo a transcatheter aortic valve replacement (TAVR). The surgical team states the patient had the procedure from a transapical approach. What is the nursing priority in her postoperative care?

    a. Hourly neurological checks

    b. Mediastinal tube patency

    c. Pain management

    d. Upper extremity neurovascular checks

27. A patient just arrived on the unit post 4-vessel Coronary Artery Bypass Graft. The surgeon reports that she used the radial artery as a conduit for the right coronary artery. She voices concern about spasm of the radial artery graft. Which of the following medications do you anticipate utilizing to reduce radial artery vasospasm?

  a. Heparin

  b. Nitroglycerin

  c. Esmolol

  d. Lisinopril

28. A 56-year-old male patient is 6 days postoperative from a CABG. He remains in the ICU for extended vasopressor needs for hypotension. Despite several attempts to wean the vasopressors, he remains on a Norepinephrine infusion. The SvO_2 reading has continually been trending down and is currently 38%. A lactate level was drawn and is now 4.8 mmol/L. He is complaining of abdominal pain and with a distended abdomen. Which postoperative complication is a concern with long-term vasopressor therapy?

  a. Splenic Infarction

  b. Ischemic Bowel

  c. Bowel Ileus

  d. Acute Tubular Necrosis

29. The nurse is caring for a patient 2 hours post cardiac surgery. The patient was placed on a spontaneous breathing trial (SBT) in preparation for extubation. The patient is breathing at a rate of 24 bpm, but denies feeling short of breath. She is able to communicate effectively by nodding and writing notes. Her skin is pink, warm & dry.

  An arterial blood gas (ABG) was obtained with the following results:

  pH 7.46

  $PaCO_2$ 32 mm Hg

PaO$_2$ 162 mm Hg

HCO$_3$ 24 mEq/L

SaO$_2$ 95%

Which intervention should the nurse anticipate?

a. Increase the set respiratory rate on the ventilator.

b. Increase the FiO$_2$.

c. Return the patient to full support settings.

d. Prepare for extubation & liberation from the ventilator.

30. During the first three hours in caring for a post-op CABG patient, the nurse observes the mediastinal chest tubes drained approximately 200 ml in the past hour. What would be the next appropriate action?

a. Continue to monitor as this is normal in the immediate post-op period

b. Elevate the head of the bed and notify the provider

c. Strip the mediastinal tubes to relieve more drainage

d. Perform an ACT test and prepare to administer protamine sulfate

31. A patient is scheduled for an elective mitral valve replacement surgery next week. He has been taking warfarin for Atrial Fibrillation. What changes to the patient's anticoagulant therapy should the nurse expect?

a. Continue to take Warfarin until the morning of the surgery

b. Stop Warfarin 1 - 2 days prior to surgery, bridge with Bivalirudin

c. Stop Warfarin 4 - 5 days prior to surgery, bridge with Heparin

d. Stop taking warfarin now

32. A 23-year-old female patient is preoperative for a mitral valve replacement due to infective endocarditis. The patient has been on antibiotic therapy for two weeks prior to surgery. The patient is a known intravenous drug user. Her urinary toxicology lab resulted positive for methamphetamines and cannabis prior to the pre-surgical care plan agreement. She rates her pain 10/10 pre-operatively. Which of the following methods of pain control might be best suitable for this patient?

a. Neurontin PO

b. Epidural

c. Percocet PO

d. NSAIDS and acetaminophen only

33. An arterial blood gas (ABG) was sent for a patient who remains intubated 12 days post 3-vessel CABG. Lung sounds are diminished in the bases and the patient has had increasing oxygen needs.

Ventilator settings:	ABG:
Assist Control mode	pH 7.28
Vt 7 ml/kg	$PaCO_2$ 55 mm Hg
Rate 20 bpm	PaO_2 62 mm Hg
FiO_2 80%	HCO_3 28 mEq/L
PEEP + 10	SaO_2 90%

A stat portable chest radiograph was ordered. Considering the blood gas results, what is the primary concern for the patient?

a. Tension pneumothorax

b. Flash pulmonary edema

c. Aspiration pneumonia

d. Acute Respiratory Distress Syndrome (ARDS)

34. A newly admitted patient post 3-vessel CABG has a Pulmonary Artery catheter in place with the following hemodynamic parameters:

HR: 116 bpm	CVP: 18 mm Hg
BP: 94/68 (77)	PA: 56/22 mm Hg
RR: 28 breaths/min	PAOP: 24 mm Hg
CO: 3.5 L/min	SV: 38 ml/beat
CI: 1.75 L/min/m²	SVR: 1896 dynes/sec/cm⁻⁵

The provider has determined the patient is in cardiogenic shock. Which of the following medications do you anticipate administering?

    a.   Digoxin and Amiodarone; the patient needs a slower heart rate.

    b.   Epinephrine and Phenylephrine; the patient needs inotropic and blood pressure support.

    c.   Crystalloids and albumin; the patient's stroke volume and preload are low and volume is needed.

    d.   Milrinone and furosemide; the patient needs a positive inotrope with vasodilator activity and a diuretic to follow.

35. Strategies which can be used to improve oxygenation include which of the following?

    a.   Increasing FiO_2 and tidal volume

    b.   Increasing tidal volume and PEEP

    c.   Decreasing set respiratory rate and PEEP

    d.   Increasing PEEP and optimizing mean airway pressure

36. A patient with a history of CAD, COPD and sudden cardiac death is scheduled for a minimally invasive CABG. Which statement from the patient regarding delirium prevention warrants additional education?

   a. "I'm so happy my wife will be able to stay the night with me."

   b. "I should be fully awake within 1 - 2 hours after the sedation medicine is stopped."

   c. "Since I will be on the ventilator longer, they will get me out of the bed while on the ventilator."

   d. "If I get agitated, they're going to give me Ativan to calm my nerves."

37. Which of the following is suggestive of Pulsus paradoxus observed with hypovolemia?

   a. Expiratory drop in SBP > 10 mm Hg

   b. Inspiratory drop in SBP > 10 mm Hg

   c. Expiratory increase in SBP > 10 mm Hg

   d. Inspiratory increase in SBP > 10 mm Hg

38. A patient who is postoperative for a left thoracotomy for a myocardial tumor removal is intubated. A spontaneous breathing trial (SBT) is being attempted. The nurse assesses labored, rapid breathing during the SBT caused from significant pain. An arterial blood gas is sent 30 minutes into the trial. Which ABG result does the nurse anticipate given the clinical presentation of the patient?

	pH	$PaCO_2$	PaO_2	HCO_3
a.	7.48	30	124	24
b.	7.45	48	138	30
c.	7.55	30	58	24
d.	7.15	70	106	18

39. A patient is 2 hours post-op CABG with bypasses to the LAD and RCA. She is in the ICU, intubated and sedated. The nurse observes jugular venous distention and the blood pressure is now 84/72 with a heart rate of 122 in sinus tachycardia. Chest tube drainage has been 100 ml for the first hour and 5 ml for the second hour. The arterial pressure waveform on the monitor shows fluctuation with breathing. Which of the following actions should be anticipated?

   a. Increase the head of bed and strip the chest tubes to promote greater drainage

   b. Notify the provider and prepare to administer a 500 ml fluid bolus

   c. Notify the provider and prepare for pericardiocentesis or resternotomy

   d. Order a STAT chest radiograph

40. A 42-year-old female patient is scheduled for an aortic valve replacement. During the pre-operative assessment, the patient states she has had consistently heavy menstrual cycles, a shoulder surgery, asthma and a tonsillectomy. The patient reports frequent epistaxis and states she bruises easily. The pre-operative RN should be most concerned about which of the following?

   a. Shoulder surgery

   b. Heavy menstrual cycles

   c. Asthma

   d. Tonsillectomy

1. The nurse is discussing pain control and management principles ith a patient and their family after cardiac surgery. Which statement y the patient demonstrates an understanding of the teaching rovided?

a. "I can expect to have no pain as I increase my activity."

b. "Effective pain control should allow me to move, walk and cough."

c. "The pain will get worse the more I walk, so I will stay in the chair."

d. "My pain goal is 0/10 pain with the pain medication."

42. Which of the following correctly describes pulse pressure?

a. Mean arterial blood pressure

b. Sum of systolic blood pressure and diastolic blood pressure

c. Difference between systolic blood pressure and diastolic blood pressure

d. Mean of systolic blood pressure and diastolic blood pressure

43. A patient with a history of Type 2 Diabetes Mellitus and chronic kidney disease (CKD) has just returned to the ICU after a 4 vessel CABG. The Anesthesiologist reports: "It was a long case and the patient received a lot of blood products."

Vital signs:	ABG results:
HR 116	pH: 7.28
BP 84/46 (59)	$PaCO_2$: 50
RR 24	PaO_2: 196
Temp 36.8°C	HCO_3: 16
	Lactate: 4.8 mmol/L

What is the nurse's primary immediate concern regarding the blood gas results?

a. Maintaining oxygenation and ventilation

b. Maintaining adequate cardiac output

c. Maintaining a negative fluid balance

d. Prevention of bleeding

44. Which of the following postoperative complications is common in almost one-third of all cardiac surgery patients?

a. Cardiac arrest postoperatively

b. Atrial Fibrillation

c. Acute Kidney Injury

d. Embolic Stroke

45. The nurse is admitting a patient post thoracic aortic aneurysm (TAA) repair with a lumbar drain in place. Which assessment finding would prompt immediate intervention from the nurse?

a. 25 mL clear CSF drainage in the lumbar drain for one hour.

b. Slight pink tinged CSF drainage visible in the drain tubing.

c. The patient unable to lift their legs off the bed or wiggle toes.

d. MAP 82 and lumbar drain pressure of 10 mm Hg by the transducer.

46. Which statement by the patient regarding postoperative extubation warrants follow up education?

a. "I can go home sooner if the breathing tube comes out within 8 hours."

b. "If there are complications during surgery, I may be on the breathing machine longer than 24 hours."

c. "I won't have pain when the tube comes out."

d. "Since I smoke, I may not qualify for early extubation."

47. A trauma patient in a high-speed collision arrives intubated to the ICU from the Emergency Department. On assessment, the patient has weak pulses in all extremities, coarse breath sounds in the bilateral bases. There is also significant bruising visible on the chest and back.

Admission vital signs are as follows:

HR 130

BP (L UE) 112/62 (78)

BP (R UE) 78/40 (53)

RR 12

T 36.0° C

Which injury does the nurse suspect?

a. Tension pneumothorax

b. Cardiac tamponade

c. Aortic dissection

d. Cardiac contusion

48. You are discussing postoperative care with your patient who is recovering from the MAZE procedure. The wife has concerns that her husband is still in Atrial Fibrillation and is requesting further information regarding future care management. Which of the following statements would be appropriate?

a. "Your husband may always be in Atrial Fibrillation, that surgery has a low success rate."

b. "That's normal for at least 6 months, check back if it persists after 6 months."

c. "If Atrial Fibrillation continues after 3 months, they will attempt cardioversion."

d. "That's normal, he'll be on amiodarone and warfarin indefinitely."

49. A 72-year-old male is 4 hours post 2-vessel CABG. Chest tube drainage was initially 30 - 60 mL/hr. For the past hour, there has been no drainage from the mediastinal chest tubes. The RN notes the following vital signs:

HR 120 bpm

BP 72/64 (66) mm Hg

CVP 20 mm Hg

PAP 60/40 mm Hg

PAOP 22 mm Hg

C.O. 3.0 L/min

C.I. 1.6 L/min/m^2

Based on the information provided, which of the following complications of cardiac surgery is suspected and requires immediate intervention?

a. Cardiogenic Shock

b. Biventricular Heart Failure

c. Myocardial Stunning

d. Cardiac Tamponade

50. A patient has just been extubated after cardiac surgery. His wife states: "I'm glad he was able to get the tube out. We were worried because this is his first surgery since he was diagnosed with obstructive sleep apnea." What would be the best immediate response?

   a. "Does he have a CPAP machine that you can bring in?"

   b. "No one told us that. I'll update his medical record now."

   c. "I can imagine your concern. We will monitor his oxygen saturation closely."

   d. "For increased safety, we will use capnography to monitor his ventilation."

51. Your patient has post-operative confusion and pulls at their Pulmonary Artery catheter. The Pulmonary Artery waveform has changed and the patient is now experiencing ventricular ectopy. The PA pressure is reading 22/6 mm Hg. Where is the catheter likely positioned and what should be done?

   a. Placement is unchanged; continue to monitor.

   b. Placement is in permanent wedge position; prepare to withdraw the catheter.

   c. Placement is in the right ventricle; prepare to withdraw the catheter back until it is in the superior vena cava or right atrium.

   d. Placement is unchanged; inflate the balloon to change the waveform.

52. The nurse is caring for a patient in the maintenance phase of the Targeted Temperature Management (TTM) protocol post cardiac arrest. The current core temperature is 33.1 °C. The nurse observes an increase in ventricular ectopy on the bedside monitor. Which electrolyte imbalance does the nurse suspect?

a. Hypokalemia & Hypomagnesemia

b. Hypermagnesemia & Hyperkalemia

c. Hypernatremia & Hyperkalemia

d. Hypophosphatemia & Hyponatremia

53. Your patient has just arrived on the unit post 3-vessel CABG. Which of the following may contribute to a prolonged ventilation?

a. Use of deep hypothermic cardiac arrest

b. Phrenic nerve injury

c. Use of Heparin with cardiopulmonary bypass

d. Severe pain requiring frequent analgesia

54. A patient is 6 hours post-op from a surgical aortic valve replacement (AVR) and the following rhythm is displayed on the monitor:

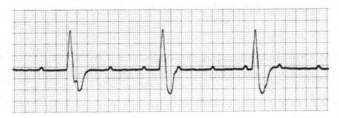

The ventricular rate is 32 bpm and the blood pressure has dropped precipitously. What is your next action?

a. Assess vital signs and prepare for epicardial pacing

b. Administer Epinephrine 0.5 mg IVP

c. Administer Atropine 0.5 mg IVP

d. Initiate an Epinephrine infusion

55. The nurse is admitting a patient to the ICU from the OR after a prolonged cardiopulmonary bypass time. The patient is intubated with epicardial pacing wires and a pulmonary artery catheter in place. The patient is on an Epinephrine (Adrenaline) infusion.

Patient data on arrival:

HR 48	CI 1.8 L/min/m^2
BP 80/42 (55) mm Hg	SVR 1720 dynes/sec/cm^{-5}
T 35.8° C	Chest tube output 50 ml
RR 14 (set)	Urine output 75 ml

What should be the priority in managing the acute hypotension?

a. Epicardial pace at a rate of 80 bpm

b. Send stat labs to assess for a coagulopathy and acidosis

c. Initiate rewarming

d. Increase the Epinephrine dose

56. Which statement by the patient indicates a need for additional education regarding post-extubation care after cardiac surgery?

a. "I will use the incentive spirometer when I get short of breath."

b. "I will use a pillow to splint my chest incision when I cough or sneeze."

c. "I will be eager to get out of the bed to prevent pneumonia."

d. "High flow oxygen by nasal cannula may decrease the risk of the tube going back in."

57. Protamine should be avoided in patients with which of the following allergies?

    a. Eggs

    b. Gluten

    c. Fish

    d. Nuts

58. A 72-year-old male patient is experiencing post-operative bleeding after cardiac surgery. Mediastinal chest tubes are draining 100 - 150 mL/hour of blood. Stat coagulation labs are obtained and reveal the following:

Hemoglobin 8.3 g/dL

Hematocrit 25%

PTT 36 seconds

PT 13.9 seconds

INR 1.1

Platelet 168 thousand/uL

Fibrinogen 80 mg/dL

The RN should anticipate administration of which of the following?

    a. Packed Red Blood Cells

    b. Platelets

    c. Fresh Frozen Plasma (FFP)

    d. Cryoprecipitate

59. You receive a patient from the ED with a BP 235/140. The patient is complaining of a headache, acute back pain, nausea, and vomiting for the past 48 hours. There is concern for aortic dissection. According to the 2017 hypertension guidelines, which of the following medications is recommended for hypertensive emergencies?

   a. Nitroglycerin

   b. Labetalol

   c. Hydralazine

   d. Nifedipine

60. A conduction defect characterized by cycles in which the PR interval progressively lengthens until a QRS complex is dropped is called:

   a.   Sinus block

   b.   Second Degree AV Block, Type I

   c.   Second Degree AV Block, Type II

   d.   Third Degree AV Block

61. The nurse is caring for an intubated patient, 2 hours after cardiac surgery. The monitor alarms with the following rhythm:

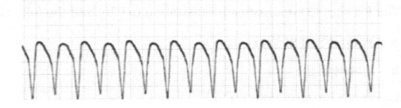

   There is no pulsatile waveform on arterial line, the patient is non-responsive and the nurse cannot palpate a femoral pulse. What should be the priority in treating this rhythm?

a.   Begin CPR until the defibrillator is ready.

b.   Activate a Code Blue response and prepare Magnesium Sulfate.

c.   Administer Lidocaine 100 mg IVP.

d.   Stimulate a cough by suctioning the patient.

62. A postoperative patient returns to the unit with an intra-aortic balloon pump (IABP). On initial assessment the patient's left radial pulse is absent. The left arm is cooler than the right. Which of the following actions should be anticipated?

a.   The balloon catheter has migrated to the subclavian artery obstructing blood flow; obtain a stat chest radiograph.

b.   The balloon catheter has migrated to the renal arteries obstructing blood flow; obtain a stat abdominal radiograph.

c.   The patient might still be cold from the Operating Room; cover the patient with warm blankets or a forced air warmer.

d.   This is a standard finding; continue to monitor the patient.

63. A 56-year-old male is admitted s/p endovascular repair of a thoracic aortic aneurysm. Approximately eight hours postoperative the patient develops bilateral lower extremity weakness and numbness.

The primary concern for this finding is:

a.   Side effects from anesthesia

b.   Positioning during the OR case

c.   Compression of the spinal arteries

d.   Baseline peripheral vascular disease

64. You are caring for a 72-year-old male immediate post-op from an aortic valve replacement secondary to severe aortic stenosis. The patient received 2 liters of Plasmalyte-A and 500 ml of cell saver blood and is currently on Norepinephrine at 0.02 mcg/kg/min and an insulin infusion at 3 units/hr.

Hemodynamic numbers upon arrival to unit:

HR 115 bpm	PAP 25/11 mm Hg
ABP 82/68 (63) mm Hg	PAOP 6 mm Hg
Cardiac Index (CI) 1.9 L/min/m²	SVR 1970 dynes/sec/cm⁻⁵
Stroke Volume Index (SVI) 23 mL/beat/m²	RVSWI 2.5 g/m²/beat
CVP 3 mm Hg	LVSWI 22 g/m²/beat

Which of the following do you anticipate as an initial intervention to treat the hemodynamic instability?

a. Administer an IV fluid bolus

b. Increase the Norepinephrine infusion dose

c. Start a Dobutamine infusion

d. Start a Phenylephrine infusion

65. A 58-year-old female post 3-vessel CABG experiences sudden cardiac arrest. Upon successful resuscitation, a 12 Lead ECG is completed. The patient's history is significant for coronary artery disease, dyslipidemia and hypertension.

This is the post-arrest 12-Lead ECG:

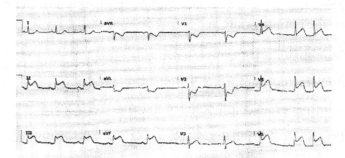

Which type of myocardial infarction is depicted on the 12-Lead ECG?

a. Anteroseptal

b. Anteroseptal-lateral

c. Inferior-lateral

d. Inferior-posterior-lateral

66. The nurse is caring for a patient status post cardiac surgery with a radial artery graft. In addition to Nitroglycerin, which medication does the nurse anticipate to prevent arterial vasospasm?

a. Morphine IV push

b. Diltiazem IV infusion

c. Amiodarone IV bolus

d. Metoprolol IV push

7. Immediately after arrival to the Cardiothoracic ICU from single-vessel CABG to the LAD and an aortic valve replacement (AVR), the nurse observes the following rhythm on the monitor:

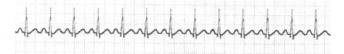

Arterial blood pressure is 156/74. The nurse questions the patient regarding the presence of pain, but the patient is still sleepy. What is your next appropriate action?

a.   Administer analgesia

b.   Administer metoprolol 5 mg IV

c.   Administer a 500 ml bolus of Lactated Ringers IV

d.   Prepare to administer digoxin (Lanoxin) 0.125 mg IV

68. A nurse is examining her 78-year-old male postoperative from a mitral valve replacement. The patient remains intubated and sedated with Propofol and Fentanyl. The patient has been hemodynamically stable. The RN has not observed movement of the patient during his 3-hour postoperative period. The RN should:

a.   Obtain an order for a STAT CT scan of the head

b.   Hold the Propofol infusion

c.   Check the patient's pupil size and responsiveness

d.   Administer Mannitol IVPB

69. You are caring for a 48-year-old male just admitted with a Type B aortic dissection. Aggressive management of blood pressure is usually accomplished with which of the following medication?

a.   Norepinephrine infusion

b.   Esmolol 50 - 200 mcg/kg/min infusion

c.   Diltiazem 5 - 15 mg/hour infusion

d.   Lisinopril 10 – 40 mg PO daily

70. The nurse is caring for a patient admitted to the ICU after a mitral valve replacement (MVR) with ventricular epicardial wires in place. Dobutamine (Dobutrex) is infusing at 10 mcg/kg/min.

Vital signs are as follows:

HR   102 (sinus tachycardia)

BP   108/64 (79) mm Hg

T   36.7° C

RR   18

SpO$_2$ 98%

The nurse should closely monitor for which of the following complications after a mitral valve replacement?

a.   Papillary muscle rupture

b.   Decreased preload

c.   Increased afterload

d.   Heart block

71. A patient is 4 hours postoperative from a mitral valve replacement. Dobutamine is infusing at 2.5 mcg/kg/min. The patient is drowsy, skin is cool to touch with some peripheral mottling noted.

The patient's hemodynamics are as follows:

HR: 72 bpm	CVP: 8 mm Hg
BP: 102/38 (59)	PAP: 65/25 mm Hg
CO: 3.9 L/min	PAOP: 12 mm Hg
CI: 1.65 L/min/m²	SVR: 2108 dynes/sec/cm⁻⁵
SV: 56 ml/beat	

Which of the following actions should be prioritized?

a. Administer crystalloids IV bolus

b. Administer Lasix 40 mg IV & initiate a norepinephrine infusion

c. Administer the scheduled metoprolol & an additional Lasix 40 mg IV

d. Increase the Dobutamine infusion to 5 mcg/kg/min and reassess the hemodynamics in 15 minutes

72. You are conducting pre-operative education for a 63-year-old female that is scheduled for open heart surgery using radial artery grafting. Which finding in the patient's social history warrants provider notification?

a. Weekly medical marijuana use

b. Plays the organ at church every Sunday

c. Teaches Pilates at the local gym

d. Volunteers at the animal shelter walking dogs

73. A patient is two days post open heart surgery. The nurse notes a sudden rhythm change on the bedside monitor to a rapid irregular heart rate. The patient is lightheaded and sweaty.

Patient vital signs are as follows:

HR 170 and irregular with a narrow QRS complex

BP 78/32 (47) mm Hg

RR 30

SpO_2 91%

Which urgent order does the nurse anticipate?

a. Amiodarone 150 mg IV bolus over 10 minutes

b. Metoprolol 10 mg IV Push

c. Adenosine 6 mg IV Push

d. Synchronized cardioversion

74. Eighteen hours after open heart surgery for mitral valve repair, a 69-year old male goes for an assisted walk with the Physical Therapy assistant. The patient experiences moderate fatigue upon returning to the chair in the room. Shortly after connecting the patient to the bedside monitor, the following rhythm is displayed:

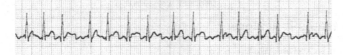

The patient denies pain or shortness of breath that is unusual for exercise. The heart rate is 172 bpm & blood pressure is 92/58 mm Hg. After getting a 12 Lead ECG, what is your next action?

a. Assist the patient back to bed, call for help and prepare for cardioversion

b. Prepare to administer Amiodarone 150 mg IV over 10 minutes

c. Prepare to administer Adenosine 6 mg rapid IV push

d. Prepare to administer Cardizem (diltiazem) 0.25 mg/kg IV push, then an infusion at 5 – 10 mg/hour

75. A patient post open heart surgery remains intubated and on the ventilator. The nurse is working to determine the appropriateness of a spontaneous breathing trial. On assessment, the patient is minimally sedated, opens eyes and follows commands.

The arterial blood gas (ABG) results:

pH 7.30

$PaCO_2$ 55 mm Hg

PaO_2 80 mm Hg

HCO_3 26 mEq/L

The nurse interprets these results as which of the following acid-base imbalance?

a.   Metabolic acidosis

b.   Metabolic alkalosis

c.   Respiratory acidosis

d.   Respiratory alkalosis

76. You receive report from the OR regarding a patient post 5-vessel Coronary Artery Bypass Graft. The patient is intubated, has AV pacing wires, 1 pleural and 2 mediastinal chest tubes, a bladder catheter and a right radial arterial line in place.

The initial hemodynamics are as follows:

HR 52 (sinus bradycardia)	PAP 32/14 mm Hg
BP 84/60 (66) mm Hg	PAOP 12 mm Hg
CI 2.0 L/min/m^2	SVR 900 dynes/sec/cm^{-5}
Stroke Volume Index (SVI) 35 mL/beat/m^2	RVSWI 7 g/m^2/beat
	LVSWI 29 g/m^2/beat
CVP 10 mm Hg	

Given the hemodynamics, which of the following should be your first intervention?

a.   Start a Dobutamine infusion

b.   Give 1000 mL IV bolus of lactated ringers

c.   Initiate atrial pacing at rate of 80 beats/min

d.   Start Phenylephrine

77. Upon assessment of a patient 3 hours post-op for CABG to RCA, LAD, and left circumflex, you observe the following: CVP is 22 mm Hg, BP 80/68 (72), chest drainage output is 20 ml total and the neck veins are distended with head of the bed at 30 degrees.

What is your next action?

a.   Notify the provider and prepare for pericardiocentesis

b.   Notify the provider and prepare for chest needle decompression

c.   Obtain STAT ABG, ionized calcium level and chest radiograph

d.   Position the head of bed flat

78. A patient with chronic kidney disease (CKD) is admitted to the ICU post open-heart surgery. The patient is intubated and sedated.

Current ventilator settings:

AMV mode

Set rate 20

Vt 10 ml/kg

FiO_2 40%

PEEP +5

Arterial blood gas (ABG) results:

pH   7.51

$PaCO_2$ 32 mm Hg

PaO_2 60 mm Hg

HCO_3 28 mEq/L

SaO_2 95%

Which intervention should the nurse anticipate?

   a.   Nephrology consultation for continuous renal replacement therapy (CRRT).

   b.   1 Liter lactated ringers bolus.

   c.   Increase the set respiratory rate and tidal volume on the ventilator.

   d.   Decrease the set respiratory rate and tidal volume on the ventilator.

79. During the bedside handoff, the OR team reports that cardiopulmonary bypass time was 5 hours. What is the most important priority the RN should anticipate as part of the immediate post-operative care?

   a.   Administration of multiple blood products

   b.   Enhanced diuresis from volume administration during surgery

   c.   Glucose resistance requiring an insulin infusion

   d.   Volume resuscitation and vasopressors to maintain the MAP

80. Which of the following is an indication for surgery in patients with mitral stenosis?

   a.   Atrial Fibrillation

   b.   Chest pain with exercise

   c.   Worsening pulmonary hypertension

   d.   Mitral valve area > 1.0 cm

81. The nurse is preparing a patient for a MAZE procedure. Which statement by the patient confirms a correct understanding of the procedure?

   a. "I will be able to leave the hospital in 2 days."

   b. "This is a minimally invasive surgery and they will enter in through the groin."

   c. "This will eventually stop my irregular heart rhythm. Scar tissue does not conduct electrical signals."

   d. "I won't have to worry about developing blood clots after this surgery anymore."

82. A 75-year-old male was difficult to wean from cardiopulmonary bypass after a 2 vessel CABG. He returns to the ICU on intra-aortic balloon counterpulsation therapy. The patient is in sinus rhythm. Two hours after his return to the unit, the nurse observes the following rhythm on the monitor:

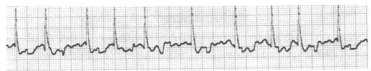

The augmented MAP from the IABP is 68 mm Hg and the heart rate is 86 bpm. The patient remains sedated on Propofol at 5 mcg/kg/min. What should be the next anticipated action?

   a. Continue to monitor the patient and ensure proper timing of the IABP

   b. Place the balloon pump in STANDBY mode and notify the surgeon

   c. Prepare to administer Amiodarone 300 mg IVP

   d. Prepare to administer Cardizem (diltiazem) 0.25 mg/kg IVP and then initiate an infusion at 5 mg/hour

83. Which patient is most appropriate for consideration of the MAZE procedure?

    a.   A tachy-dysrhythmia requiring a permanent pacemaker

    b.   Atrial Fibrillation refractory to medication

    c.   Supportive of tricuspid valve replacement

    d.   Atrial septal defect repair

84. Which of the following correctly describes the characteristics of a pericardial friction rub auscultated in pericarditis after a myocardial infarction?

    a.   Harsh and intermittent sound

    b.   Low pitched rumbling sound

    c.   High pitched blowing sound

    d.   Scratchy sound like Velcro

85. A 65-year-old female presents to the ED with a complaint of retrosternal chest pain. History is significant for hypercholesterolemia, dyslipidemia, hypertension, inferior wall MI and chronic Atrial Fibrillation. The patient is admitted with NSTE-ACS and a 3 vessel CABG is scheduled. The surgeon desires to use the left radial artery as a graft.

Which of the following would be a contraindication of using the radial artery as a graft as planned?

    a.   Negative Allen's test on the left extremity

    b.   Negative Allen's test on the right extremity

    c.   Positive Allen's test on the left extremity

    d.   Positive Allen's test on the right extremity

86. A patient is complaining of sudden onset chest pain and palpitations. The monitor shows paroxysmal supraventricular tachycardia (PSVT) with a ventricular rate of 190 beats/min. If vagal maneuvers are unsuccessful, which medication should you anticipate to administer?

    a. Amiodarone

    b. Esmolol

    c. Adenosine

    d. Digoxin

87. A 54-year-old diabetic patient returns to the Cardiac Surgery clinic six days after discharge from the hospital from a 2-vessel CABG. The RN is assessing the patient and asking about the patient's diet, exercise, and general well-being. The RN should be most concerned about which statement from the patient?

    a. "I have been walking to get the mail every day."

    b. "I have been eating a lot of spinach in my smoothies each morning."

    c. "I have been checking my blood glucose and using more insulin than I normally do."

    d. "I have lost about 4 pounds since surgery."

88. The nurse is admitting a patient to the ICU with an aortic dissection that begins in the ascending aorta and extends near the iliac arteries. The patient is at significant risk of stroke, heart failure and death. The nurse understands the patient's priority plan includes:

    a. Immediate surgery for repair.

    b. Endovascular repair procedure with stent.

    c. Medical management with vasodilators.

    d. Nothing unless the aneurysm ruptures.

89. On post-op day #2 after a CABG, the patient is extubated. At 1700, the patient becomes agitated and uncooperative. Upon questioning, the patient's partner states: "He drinks 2 - 5 vodka martinis a day." What should the nurse anticipate next?

   a. Administration of Ativan (lorazepam) 1 mg IVP

   b. Immediate intubation and continuous infusion of Propofol IV

   c. Perform the CIWA assessment and notify the provider

   d. Perform delirium assessment and notify the provider

90. The nurse is precepting a new nurse in the care of a patient post thoracic aortic aneurysm (TAA) repair. Which statement by the new nurse demonstrates an understanding of the risks associated with the surgical procedure?

   a. "Cross clamping the aorta directly increases blood flow to the kidneys."

   b. "Cross clamping the aorta can impact perfusion to the spinal cord."

   c. "Abdominal aneurysms have no risk of paralysis."

   d. "Bleeding is a low risk postoperatively."

Answers Practice Exam 1

1. A. Incentive spirometry. Atelectasis is one of the most common complications post-surgery and is recognized by diminished lung sounds with basilar crackles and increasing oxygen needs. Nursing priorities should focus on prevention of atelectasis including incentive spirometry, coughing and deep breathing and mobility. Increasing the chest tube suction will not improve oxygenation or lung expansion. Crackles noted in the bilateral bases would improve with alveolar expansion, improved gas exchange and coughing and deep breathing. BiPAP may be necessary if respiratory distress is present and gas exchange continues to worsen, which can include CO_2 retention. However, it is not appropriate at this point.

2. C. Obesity. Deep sternal wound infections may occur in approximately in 1 - 4% of postoperative patients and carries a mortality rate of up to 25%. Adipose is avascular and antibiotics are poorly distributed. Another high-risk patient population includes patients who have both the left and right internal mammary arteries used as grafts. The internal mammary arteries perfuse the chest wall. Using both mammary arteries for grafting may increase the risk of sternal wound infection.

3. C. Bleeding. Bleeding in the postoperative period is frequently related to the coagulopathic effect of extracorporeal circulation during cardiopulmonary bypass. This can be attributed to impaired coagulation due to hepatic congestion associated with end stage heart failure and treatment with anticoagulants. Although von Willebrand Syndrome can be acquired in these patients, it typically develops more than a week post device implantation. Drive line infections can also occur after device implantation. GI obstruction was more common with the pulsatile first-generation devices inserted into the abdomen, but is rare with axial flow pumps not implanted in the abdomen.

4. D. Complete heart block. According to the Transcatheter Valve Therapy (TVT) registry, approximately 8 - 43% of all patients following the TAVR procedure therapy will require a permanent pacemaker due to developing heart block within the first 30 days. Those patients who receive the self-expanding CoreValve have a higher rate of pacemaker implantation when compared to the balloon expandable valve. New onset atrial fibrillation is seen in about 6% of all TAVR cases.

5. A. Desmopressin. In von Willebrand's Type I disease, desmopressin stimulates the release of von Willebrand's factor from endothelial cells, which increases the coagulant factor by 3 to 5-fold. Norepinephrine may treat the patient's hypotension, but would have no effect on bleeding or the effects of von Willebrand's disease. The reversal of coagulopathy & bleeding should be a primary focus in treatment.

6. B. Decreased cardiac index, increased SVR, increased PAOP, increased CVP. Due to ineffective pumping of the ventricle, the cardiac output decreases while PAOP and CVP/preload increase. Because of decreased perfusion to organs, the sympathetic nervous system is activated to increase perfusion by vasoconstricting to shunt blood from the periphery to the core. The result is increased systemic vascular resistance or afterload.

7. D. Increased filling pressures, decreased cardiac output, narrow pulse pressure. Tamponade can occur with uncontrolled bleeding accumulating in the pericardium or from clotted mediastinal chest tubes. Tamponade should be suspected if there is a sudden drop or cessation in previously significant mediastinal bleeding. Signs of tamponade include: rising filling pressures (CVP & PAOP), decreased cardiac output, hypotension, narrowed pulse pressure, tachycardia, muffled heart tones, JVD, dysrhythmias, decreased ECG voltage and widened mediastinum on chest x-ray.

8. C. Assess the quality of compressions. Capnography during resuscitation is used as a marker of perfusion and assessment of the return of spontaneous circulation (ROSC). Waveform capnography is reflective of perfusion and transport of CO_2 to the lungs. If the data provided is demonstrating that perfusion is poor, then compression quality needs to be assessed and improved.

Normal exhaled carbon dioxide ($PEtCO_2$) is 35 - 45 mm Hg. A $PEtCO_2$ < 10 mm Hg may signify a need for an improvement in compression quality. A rapid increase in $PEtCO_2$ may clinically indicate ROSC. A prolonged time with a $PEtCO_2$ < 10 mm Hg in the setting of high-quality CPR should prompt a team discussion of termination of resuscitation, especially if the rhythm terminates to asystole. An exception to this is a pulmonary embolism. If a PE is the cause of the arrest, the $PEtCO_2$ value may be consistently low.

9. C. Leaflet fibrosis and retraction occurs with repair, leading to aortic regurgitation. Debridement of aortic valve calcification often results in early postoperative atrial regurgitation from leaflet fibrosis and retraction, a process that progresses over time.

10. D. Meticulous sternal incision care. Use of bilateral internal mammary arteries pose an increased risk of sternal wound infections. The internal mammary arteries perfuse the chest wall and sternum. Maintenance and care of the sternal incision is of high importance to improve patient outcomes and prevent infection. Pulmonary toileting will be a priority with all post CABG patients regardless of the graft used.

11. A. Furosemide (Lasix) 40 mg IVP. The patient is demonstrating signs of Transfusion Associated Circulatory Overload (TACO). Dyspnea/orthopnea, peripheral & pulmonary edema and rapid increase in blood pressure are hallmark signs of this condition. TACO responds well to diuretic therapy. Continuing the transfusion will only add circulating volume making the situation worse. A second vasodilator will treat the symptom of the issue, but not correct the problem. Increasing the PEEP may correct the SpO_2 and PaO_2 levels however; it can further reduce cardiac output by decreasing venous return.

12. A. Reduced risk of bleeding. The avoidance of cardiopulmonary bypass (CPB) with off-pump CABG has advantages over on-pump CABG. These include decreased risk for bleeding, decreased anemia & need for transfusions and decreased risk of AKI. In addition, the patient should be kept normothermic to prevent arrhythmias, bleeding, vasoconstriction and postoperative shivering.

13. B. One liter of lactated ringers IV bolus. The patient is showing signs of decreased cardiac output related to hypovolemia. Vasopressor administration without adequate fluid volume resuscitation can potentially worsen cardiac output. Blood is not indicated as the patient is demonstrating hypovolemia not related to bleeding as evidenced by the lab values. Chest tube output is not indicative of increased bleeding.

14. B. Acute ventricular septal rupture. A new onset murmur following an Anteroseptal myocardial infarction, coupled with an acute elevation in pulmonary artery pressure are classic findings of a post infarction ventricular septal rupture. Septal ruptures after a MI are not as common now as they were in the pre-fibrinolytic era, but if they are seen, it is typically 3 to 8 days following a MI. Left ventricular free wall rupture is also possible, but usually presents as severe chest pain and can deteriorate to cardiac arrest. Mitral valve prolapse is also possible following a MI, but would not cause an abrupt increase in pulmonary artery pressures.

15. A. Hypocalcemia, hypokalemia, hypomagnesemia, hypophosphatemia. All of the aforementioned electrolytes can be deficient after cardiac surgery. The exception may be potassium; hypo or hyperkalemia may be present. Causes of electrolyte deficiencies following cardiac surgery are multifactorial. Often, hypokalemia, hypocalcemia, hypomagnesemia, and hypophosphatemia result from hemodilution after cardiopulmonary bypass, especially with the use of electrolyte free solutions, diuretic usage, administration of banked blood, treatment of hyperglycemia, and hypothermia. Alternatively, hyperkalemia may be present as a result of the cardioplegia solution used during bypass, metabolic acidosis, hemolysis of red blood cells or renal dysfunction.

16. C. Increasing the Epinephrine infusion for hypotension. Patients should be weaned and assessed with a spontaneous breathing trial as soon as they are awake and following commands, hemodynamically stable, have minimal chest tube drainage and appropriate ABG values. Signs of weaning failure include: agitation, increased respiratory rate, SpO_2 < 90%, diaphoresis or accessory muscle use, tachycardia and an increasing need for vasopressor or inotropic support.

17. B. CI 1.9 L/min/m^2, CVP 2 mm Hg, PAOP 6 mm Hg, HR 120. In the setting of hypovolemia related to hemorrhage, the nurse should anticipate seeing a drop in cardiac output as evidenced by a decrease in stroke volume with a decrease in preload (CVP/PAOP). A subsequent increase in the heart rate is a compensatory response to the decrease in stroke volume. An increase in preload/right atrial pressure (CVP) or pulmonary artery occlusive pressure (PAOP) would not be expected and would likely be observed with fluid overload.

18. A. Assess and treat pain. During the immediate postoperative period, pain management is a priority. The patient may still be under the effects of anesthesia and subsequently may be unable to respond to verbal inquiries. Pain and/or agitation may be an underlying cause of the hypertension. If the blood pressure remains elevated after the administration of pain medication, a vasodilating medication like Nitroglycerin may be administered via intravenous infusion.

19. A. Synchronized Cardioversion. Cardioversion is indicated in a patient experiencing new onset atrial fibrillation who is unstable with symptomatic hypotension. If the patient was normotensive, medications would be considered for rate or rhythm control.

20. A. Return the patient to their original position. The transvenous wire may have migrated & dislodged with the position change. By returning the patient to their original supine position, the potential for the lead to come in contact with myocardial tissue and pace is increased. The patient may also benefit from being placed on their left side to float the wire toward the right ventricular septum. If pacing does not resume, the nurse should prepare to transcutaneous pace the patient until the wire can be repositioned.

21. C. Anemia. Often patients will experience anemia with Cardiopulmonary Bypass surgery. Transfusion thresholds in this patient have been explored. In 2017, published in the New England Journal of Medicine - Transfusion Requirements in Cardiac Surgery (TRICS) investigators identified that a restrictive red blood cell transfusion strategy (Hgb < 7.5 g/dL) was noninferior to a conservative strategy (Hgb < 9.0 g/dL). On average 30% of all patients who undergo CABG require red blood cell transfusion. Renal failure, mediastinitis and graft failure are all complications, but their incidences are lower than blood transfusion.

22. C. Vasopressin. Vasoplegic vasodilation can occur in the setting of prolonged CPB time secondary to leukocyte activation, release of pro-inflammatory mediators and nitric oxide production by endothelial cells. Vasoplegic syndrome, characterized by low arterial pressure with normal or elevated cardiac index and reduced systemic vascular resistance, occurs in 5% - 25% of patients undergoing cardiac surgery.

Refractory hypotension that occurs in the presence of adequate filling pressures and preserved pump function, is commonly secondary to a failure to respond to catecholamines, also known as catecholamine resistance.

In severe Vasoplegic states, vascular smooth muscle cells may become unresponsive to norepinephrine because of complex mechanisms that include activation of adenosine triphosphate–sensitive K^+ channels, increased nitric oxide synthesis, adrenoceptor desensitization, and vasopressin and corticosteroid deficiency.

Consideration should be given to adding an infusion of a vasopressor such vasopressin, which promotes contraction of smooth muscle cells causing peripheral vasoconstriction and increases secretion of corticotropin.

23. B. Administer diuretics for volume overload due to a history of heart failure with reduced ejection fraction. Transfusion associated circulatory overload (TACO) is the most likely cause of this patient's acute decompensation related to volume overload; thus, the most appropriate action is to administer diuretics. TACO is often under reported given that it is not transfusion-related acute lung injury (TRALI), which is often required to report. The risk of TACO increases with a history of heart failure and correlates with the number of units transfused.

TRALI is thought to be caused by activation of the recipient's neutrophils by donor antibodies and causes inflammatory acute lung injury. TRALI is different from TACO because there is an absence of circulatory overload often with a normal PAOP. If the patient responds to diuretics, that is another sign that is more consistent with TACO vs. TRALI.

24. C. Remove unnecessary invasive devices. Removing unnecessary invasive devices including urinary catheters, central lines and IVs are a vital part of the nursing plan of care to advance the patient's outcome. Minimizing invasive devices, early mobilization, and promotion of sleep and rest can minimize the risk of delirium development for individuals at the highest risk. In addition, delirium causing medications such as benzodiazepines should be avoided if possible.

25. A. Papillary Muscle Rupture. Papillary muscle rupture is a potential complication of myocardial infarctions associated with the inferior or anterior walls. Symptoms of papillary muscle rupture include a systolic murmur, hypotension, increased PAOP and reduced cardiac output. The patient will have enlarged v waves on the PAOP tracing. The goal of IABP therapy is to reduce afterload to reduce mitral regurgitation. Aortic insufficiency and thoracic aneurysms are contraindications to IABP therapy. Tricuspid stenosis is not a primary indication.

26. B. Mediastinal tube patency. Complications associated with the transapical approach to TAVR is increased risk for cardiac tamponade, pain and respiratory compromise. It is vital that mediastinal tube patency is assessed frequently to avert the possibility of cardiac tamponade.

27. B. Nitroglycerin. The radial artery is often used as a graft, but is prone to spasm because of its musculature nature. Competing blood flow through the native coronary artery reduces blood flow through the arterial graft and increases the risk for spasm and atrophy. The risk of spasm can be decreased with IV nitrates post-operatively. Often patients are transitioned to oral calcium channel blockers during hospitalization and after discharge for a short period of time.

28. B. Ischemic Bowel. Clinical signs and symptoms of an ischemic bowel include hypoactive bowel tones, abdominal distention, abdominal pain and rising lactate levels with decreasing SvO_2 levels. This patient is at risk for ischemic bowel given his prolonged need for vasopressors with hypotension. Any low cardiac output state for a prolonged period of time puts a patient at risk for developing ischemic bowel. Splenic infarctions are usually caused by thromboembolism. Pain related to acute tubular necrosis would be rare.

29. D. Prepare for extubation & liberation from the ventilator. Slight alkalosis can indicate hyperventilation on the spontaneous breathing mode. It may be clinically related to pain or breathing against resistance from the endotracheal tube, but is not a concern or risk for success post-extubation. The nurse's priority is to examine the physical assessment of the patient as well as the ABG results for evidence of hypoventilation and/or hypoxemia. That is not evident in this assessment.

30. B. Elevate the head of the bed and notify the provider. Elevating the head of the bed facilitates mediastinal tube drainage, decreases preload and decreases bleeding. Two hundred ml's of drainage in one hour is excessive. The patient is experiencing postoperative hemorrhage and potentially needs to go back to surgery. Coagulation studies as well as a STAT hemoglobin & platelets should be assessed. Notification of the provider is imperative.

31. C. Stop Warfarin 4 - 5 days prior to surgery, bridge with Heparin. Medications affecting hemostasis or bleeding, specifically warfarin, are discontinued in preparation for cardiac surgery. The terminal half-life of warfarin after a single dose is approximately 1 week; however, the effective half-life ranges from 20 to 60 hours, with a mean of about 40 hours.

The American College of Chest Physicians recommends warfarin be held 4 - 5 days prior to surgery to allow the INR to normalize to minimize the bleeding risk with surgery. They suggest IV unfractionated heparin (UFH) be used as a bridge for high-risk of thrombosis, as in the case of Atrial Fibrillation and prior embolic event, to provide prophylaxis against development of a recurrent embolism. Unfractionated heparin has a half-life of about one to two hours after infusion, whereas low-molecular-weight Heparin has a half-life about four times longer. Guidelines suggest starting intravenous UFH when the INR drops to less than 2 and to discontinue the intravenous UFH 6 hours before surgery.

32. B. Epidural. Epidural agents may be most beneficial for a patient with drug dependency. Narcotics will help to treat the patient's pain, but due to her IV drug history, it may be difficult to manage and require higher doses. Acetaminophen and oral agents will be good supplements and an option for transition once the epidural is removed. NSAIDS should be used with caution with cardiac surgery patients as they can increase the bleeding risk and cause renal dysfunction.

33. D. Acute Respiratory Distress Syndrome (ARDS). ARDS is a condition of massive inflammation in the lungs resulting in non-cardiogenic pulmonary edema, leaky pulmonary capillaries, leukocyte infiltration in the lungs, decreased pulmonary compliance (stiff lungs), and endothelial and alveolar damage.

The clinical presentation of ARDS includes tachypnea, refractory hypoxemia (worsening hypoxemia despite increases in FiO_2), and bilateral pulmonary infiltrates seen on chest x-ray. The P/F ratio is the PaO_2 divided by the fraction of inspired O_2 (FiO_2). A P/F ratio of 200 - 300 meets diagnostic criteria for mild ARDS. The P/F ratio in this case is currently 77 and meets the Berlin criteria to be categorized as severe ARDS. This significantly increases patient mortality postoperatively.

Obtaining a chest x-ray is an appropriate next step in supporting the likely diagnosis. Pneumonia is a consideration, but there is no reason to believe from the data presented that the patient aspirated. Pulmonary edema would present as coarse crackles on auscultation.

Treatment for ARDS should include lung protective ventilation strategies. This includes decreasing the tidal volume to 4 – 6 ml/kg, utilizing PEEP to improve oxygenation and keeping the plateau pressure < 30 cm H_2O, prone positioning and inhaled pulmonary vasodilators like Epoprostenol (iFlolan) or Nitric Oxide (iNO). If the patient is dysynchronous with the ventilator, neuromuscular blockade should also be considered.

34. D. Milrinone and furosemide; the patient needs a positive inotrope with vasodilator activity and a diuretic to follow. Milrinone is a positive inotrope with vasodilator effects. It will decrease the SVR and improve the cardiac output and index by promoting better forward flow. When forward flow improves, a diuretic will promote excess fluid removed likely resulting in improved pulmonary artery pressures.

35. D. Increasing PEEP and optimizing mean airway pressure. Settings on the ventilator which influence oxygenation include FiO_2 – fraction of inspired oxygen delivered to the patient and PEEP – Positive End Expiratory Pressure. PEEP maintains positive pressure in the lungs at the end of expiration and prevents alveolar collapse. This improves oxygenation and mean airway pressure. Mean airway pressure is the average airway pressure of the total ventilator cycle time. Increasing the mean airway pressure in turn increases the surface area in the lung available for oxygenation. Adjustments in tidal volume and respiratory rate will influence ventilation, which is reflected in the $PaCO_2$ and pH on an ABG.

36. D. "If I get agitated, they're going to give me Ativan to calm my nerves." Benzodiazepine administration for delirium generally does not improve patient outcomes. In fact, benzos are thought to actually contribute to delirium & make it worse. The Pain-Agitation-Delirium-Immobility-Sleep (PADIS) Guidelines should be followed to ensure delirium is ideally prevented, but identified early and treated appropriately.

37. B. Inspiratory drop in SBP > 10 mm Hg. The findings suggestive of Pulsus paradoxus include an exaggerated drop in stroke volume during breathing. Clinically, this results in a drop in the systolic BP during inspiration > 10 mm Hg. These changes are caused from increased intra-thoracic pressure causing compression of the inferior vena cava, leading to decreased venous return. Pulsus paradoxus can be observed in hypovolemia, cardiac tamponade, constrictive pericarditis, superior vena cava obstruction, airway obstruction, COPD and asthma.

38. A. pH 7.48, $PaCO_2$ 30, PaO_2 124, HCO_3 24. The nurse would anticipate a slight respiratory alkalosis from the impact of pain and rapid labored breathing. Because of the brief timing of the SBT, the nurse would not expect a change in renal compensation, a change in the serum HCO_3 or severe hypoxemia.

39. C. Notify the provider and prepare for pericardiocentesis or resternotomy. Jugular venous distention (JVD), tachycardia and hypotension with narrow pulse pressure & Pulsus paradoxus in conjunction with an abrupt decrease in mediastinal tube drainage is suspicious for cardiac tamponade. In this case the provider should be notified immediately. The nurse should prepare for pericardiocentesis or resternotomy. In addition, coagulation labs should be assessed. A chest radiograph is appropriate, but notification of the provider is the biggest priority in the setting of cardiac tamponade.

40. B. Heavy menstrual cycles. This could be a potential sign of von Willebrand Disease (vWD), which is a hereditary disease that affects the facilitation of platelet adhesion. This can result in hemorrhagic complications postoperatively. Of note, aortic valve stenosis can also cause stress on the endothelium and activate an inflammatory reaction of von Willebrand factor levels. This resolves with valve repair. Asthma is a concern regarding intubation and extubation of the patient, however, it can usually be managed with bronchodilators.

Treatment for von Willebrand's Disease includes desmopressin (DDAVP), recombinant von Willebrand Factor (rvWF) & von Willebrand factor/factor VIII concentrate. Platelet transfusions may also be helpful for Type III vWD.

41. B. "Effective pain control should allow me to move, walk and cough." Utilization of a valid pain scale is an important nursing assessment tool for evaluation of the effectiveness of pain control. However, in tailoring the pain control, it is effective if the patient is able to increase activity, mobilization, and risk reduction activities. This should be an active part of the nursing plan of care and communication in the education provided as well as documentation of evaluation of progression and recovery after surgery.

42. C. Difference between systolic blood pressure and diastolic blood pressure. Pulse pressure (PP) is defined as the difference between systolic blood pressure (SBP) and diastolic blood pressure (DBP). PP = SBP - DBP. Normal pulse pressure is about 40 mm Hg. Conditions of narrow pulse pressure include cardiac tamponade. Wide pulse pressure conditions include aortic valvular regurgitation and brain stem herniation.

43. B. Maintaining adequate cardiac output. The blood gas results reveal a combined respiratory & metabolic acidosis with an elevated lactate level. In addition to bleeding & volume loss, acidosis can have negative inotropic effects on the myocardium resulting in decreased cardiac output. Maintaining sufficient cardiac output is the priority until the acidosis is properly managed & corrected.

44. B. Atrial Fibrillation. Because the surgical intervention is within the proximity of the AV node, Atrial Fibrillation is a common complication, occurring in 20 - 40% of patients after a CABG. If a patient develops Afib, it should be treated appropriately to prevent decreased cardiac output and the potential for thromboembolism. Two approaches are common with Atrial Fibrillation management post CABG. The options are to either rate control or rhythm control. Neither have demonstrated to be superior over the other, as they are equally safe and effective.

Rate control can be done via beta blockers, calcium channel blockers or digoxin. Rhythm control can be accomplished with anti-arrhythmic medications or through electrical cardioversion. If Atrial Fibrillation persists beyond 24 – 48 hours, anticoagulation should be considered.

45. C. The patient unable to lift their legs off the bed or wiggle toes. The spine is at significant risk of ischemia after TAA repair. The lumbar drain is in place to minimize ischemia from swelling and edema following cross clamping time required during the operative repair of a TAA. Lumbar pressure goals are < 10 mm Hg, but maintaining an overall perfusion pressure > 70 (MAP – ICP = PP) is most important to the spinal cord. Paraplegia and spinal cord ischemia can occur in upwards of 25% of cases. Closely monitoring neurologic exams and responding immediately to slight decreases is the nursing priority post-surgical repair.

46. C. "I won't have pain when the tube comes out." The patient should be evaluated frequently for pain postoperatively. The nurse should communicate a pain management strategy with the patient. This will likely result in improved control of pain, expectations that are met, and an overall better experience for the patient.

47. C. Aortic dissection. Aortic injuries, shearing & dissections are a risk with traumatic acceleration/deceleration force thoracic injury. Systolic BP differences between bilateral upper extremities of > 25 mm Hg are a significant finding on assessment. The nurse should have a high level of suspicion for an aortic injury.

48. C. "If Atrial Fibrillation continues after 3 months, they will attempt cardioversion." It is not uncommon for patients to continue to have Atrial Fibrillation (A-Fib) for a few months after the MAZE procedure due to swelling, fluid changes, and relearning of electrical pathways. The patient will likely be discharged on oral Amiodarone and warfarin. If A-Fib persists after 3 months, electrical cardioversion may be attempted. If cardioversion is unsuccessful, the patient will be sent home on warfarin only. The MAZE procedure has a high success rate, with A-Fib being eliminated in 50 - 90% of patients.

49. D. Cardiac Tamponade. Hallmark symptoms are tachycardia, hypotension, narrow pulse pressure, jugular venous distention, equalization of intra-cardiac pressures and increasing filling pressures. This patient's pulse pressure is 8 mm Hg. Reminder, pulse pressure is calculated by subtracting the diastolic pressure from the systolic pressure. Normal pulse pressure is 40 mm Hg. Tamponade requires immediate surgical intervention by either pericardiocentesis or open re-sternotomy. Although all the choices provided would have a similar hemodynamic profile, the story gives an indication leading to cardiac tamponade.

50. D. "For increased safety, we will use capnography to monitor his ventilation." Patients who are opioid-naïve, especially with a history of obstructive sleep apnea are at an increased risk for opioid-induced respiratory depression due to hypoventilation. A rise in end-tidal CO_2 will be seen before changes in vital signs, including oxygen saturation. In addition, the patient's home CPAP machine may be used when he sleeps. In the meantime, Capnography should be used as a safety monitoring measure to identify hypoventilation, as evidenced by an increasing $EtCO_2$.

51. C. Placement is in the right ventricle; prepare to withdraw the catheter back until it is in the superior vena cava or right atrium. The patient has more than likely pulled the pulmonary artery catheter into the right ventricle, which can cause ectopy and potential arrhythmias. Pull the catheter back, and either prepare to discontinue it, or have a provider advance it to the pulmonary artery.

52. A. Hypokalemia & Hypomagnesemia. A side effect of Targeted Temperature Management during the cooling phase (32 – 34° C) is hypokalemia, hypomagnesemia and hypophosphatemia. The effects of electrolyte shifting are most significant during the cooling and early rewarming phases. Cardiac dysrhythmias and ectopy are clinical indicators of shifting electrolytes and should prompt evaluation by the nurse.

53. B. Phrenic nerve injury. Cold cardioplegic solution can cause damage to the diaphragm and injury to the phrenic nerve. On chest radiograph this may be seen by an elevated diaphragm. Effects on the diaphragm may cause respiratory compromise, atelectasis & prolonged ventilation. This may require a tracheostomy for prolonged support and slower weaning.

The use of deep hypothermic arrest is used in most cardiothoracic cases, therefore does not specifically cause prolonged ventilation in this patient population unless the circulatory arrest time is significantly prolonged. Prolonged cross clamping of the descending aorta can result in hypoperfusion, paraplegia, or renal failure. The large incisions can be very painful, but judicious use of analgesia therapy should not delay extubation.

54. A. Assess vital signs and prepare for epicardial pacing. Epicardial wires are routinely placed after valve surgery. For third degree AV block, the patient's hemodynamic status should be evaluated and the nurse should prepare for epicardial pacing using the ventricular wires exiting the chest from the left of the sternum and atrial wires from the right. DDD pacing mode would be the most desirable mode, where both the atria & ventricles are paced & sensed with an inhibition to pacing if the patient has intrinsic competition.

If epicardial wires were not placed, the patient can be transcutaneous paced, transitioning to transvenous pacing. In complete heart block, atropine is often not effective as is accelerates the SA node rate. Epinephrine may cause a significant increase in the ventricular rate, leading to demand ischemia. Emergent pacing would be the initial therapy.

55. A. Epicardial pace at a rate of 80 bpm. Components of cardiac output are heart rate and stroke volume. Bradycardia is anticipated post-cardiac surgery. The initial priority is to ensure that cardiac output needs are being met. Increasing the heart rate via epicardial pacing to increase the cardiac output is the first priority intervention by the nurse. Epinephrine may also be increased, however that would increase the patient's SVR and afterload, which is already elevated. This may increase the workload of the heart.

56. A. "I will use the incentive spirometer when I get short of breath." The patient will require a strict regimen for use of the incentive spirometer (IS) to prevent atelectasis. Utilization of the IS every hour while awake for 10 reps is a typical recommendation post-operative from thoracic surgery. All of the other statements are appropriate.

57. C. Fish. Protamine is derived from salmon sperm. Patients with allergies to fish may be at risk for anaphylaxis. Treatment of anaphylaxis includes Epinephrine (1:1000) 0.3 mg IM, histamine blockers; Benadryl (H1) & Pepcid or Ranitidine (H2). Steroids may also be considered.

58. D. Cryoprecipitate. Cryoprecipitate is indicated as key replacement factor because the patient has a low fibrinogen. If the patient continues to bleed, exploratory reoperation may be needed. The patient may also receive FFP or platelets if bleeding continues with a dropping platelet count or increased INR.

59. B. Labetalol. The primary goal is to determine which patients with acute hypertension are exhibiting symptoms of end-organ damage and require immediate intravenous (IV) therapy. An added benefit of labetalol is the beta blocking actions will also slow the heart rate, which a desired goal in a suspected aortic dissection. In aortic dissection, the preferred medications are labetalol, nicardipine, nitroprusside, esmolol, and morphine sulfate. The goal is to rapidly lower the SBP to target of 100 – 110 mm Hg within 20 minutes. Then, maintain the SBP < 110 mm Hg, unless signs of end-organ hypoperfusion are present.

The preferred treatment includes a combination of narcotic analgesics (morphine sulfate), beta blockers (labetalol, esmolol), and vasodilators (nicardipine, nitroprusside). Labetalol is particularly preferred in patients with acute dissection and end-stage renal disease. Calcium channel blockers (verapamil, diltiazem) are an alternative to beta blockers. Caution should be taken, as a rapid decrease in BP can cause ischemic damage in vascular beds & organs that are used to higher pressure.

60. B. Second degree AV Block, Type I. Sinus block is characterized by a constant PR interval, not lengthening, followed by a blocked impulse. Second degree AV Block, Type II has a constant PR interval for those impulses conducted to the ventricles. Third Degree AV Block is characterized by no association or pattern to the PR interval and a regular ventricular rhythm. The ventricular rhythm originates in the ventricles, giving a wide QRS and slow ventricular rate. In Second Degree AV block, Type I, the PR interval progressively lengthens until the QRS complex is dropped. Definition: 1) Progressive prolongation of the PR interval culminating in a non-conducted P wave. 2) The PR interval is usually longest immediately before the dropped beat. 3) The PR interval is shortest immediately after the dropped beat.

61. A. Begin CPR until the defibrillator is ready. Defibrillation is the ultimate priority, but until the defibrillator can be obtained and connected, high quality CPR should be initiated without delay. The shock should be delivered as quickly as possible to terminate the rhythm.

62. A. The balloon catheter has migrated to the subclavian artery obstructing blood flow; obtain a stat chest radiograph. The balloon pump catheter, if malpositioned or dislodged, can cause perfusion problems. If the left radial pulse is absent or noticeably weaker than the right, the balloon pump may be blocking the left subclavian artery, preventing blood flow to the left arm. The first action would be to get a chest radiograph to confirm placement.

63. C. Compression of the spinal arteries. Cord ischemia can develop from compression of the spinal arteries related to swelling surrounding the graft, as well as in relation to the portion of the aorta which is covered by the graft. This is clinically significant and should be addressed immediately. Spinal cord ischemia is less common with endovascular repair vs. open repair of the aorta.

This would be a late finding for positioning from the OR case or as a side effect from anesthesia. In addition, anesthesia typically produces non-focal deficits where these are specific to the lower extremities.

64. A. Administer an IV fluid bolus. Increased HR, low SVI with a low PAOP and CVP suggest fluid administration should be the initial intervention. Patients with aortic stenosis have chronically compensated with a hyperdynamic left ventricle. Once the valve is replaced there is no longer the increased pressure the ventricle must overcome, but the ventricle has not had time to adapt. Patients often require higher filling pressures to maintain adequate cardiac output. Increasing Norepinephrine or starting Phenylephrine will increase afterload, which is already elevated and will likely lead to decreased stroke volume. Starting Dobutamine without adequate preload may worsen cardiac function.

65. D. Inferior-posterior-lateral. Leads II, III and aVF examine the inferior wall of the left ventricle. Leads V5 and V6 assess the low lateral wall of the left ventricle. In all of the aforementioned leads, there is the pattern of ST segment elevation indicative of myocardial injury. In the presence of an Inferior wall MI, ST segment depression in leads V1 and V2 with deep R-waves indicate an acute posterior wall MI. This is a reciprocal change of the posterior wall. The ST segment depression in leads I & aVL are reciprocal changes of the inferior wall infarction. This patient will require immediate revascularization.

66. B. Diltiazem IV infusion. In addition to nitroglycerin, calcium channel blockers work effectively to prevent and minimize arterial vasospasm. Arterial vasospasm can impede blood flow and contribute to development of tissue ischemia.

67. A. Administer analgesia. Immediately after surgery the patient may continue to have residual effects of any neuromuscular blocking agents (NMBAs) administered in the OR. Should the sedation effects begin to wane before those of the NMBAs, the patient may experience pain, although not visibly evident. It is appropriate in this case to administer analgesia. In sinus tachycardia rhythms, the goal is always to treat the underlying cause of the tachycardia. In this case pain is the most likely cause.

68. B. Hold the Propofol infusion. Before a neurological assessment can be performed accurately, the RN must stop sedatives that may affect the exam. A STAT CT scan of the head would be warranted after a complete neurological exam and the patient has had time to metabolize his sedative medications. Pupillary reactivity should be assessed, but are a late sign of neurological changes. Mannitol would be administered only in there was reason to believe the patient had increased intracranial pressure.

69. B. Esmolol 50 - 200 mcg/kg/min infusion. Type B dissections, or aortic dissections of the descending aorta can be considered for initial medical management with anti-hypertensives and may require surgery or stenting long term. Therefore, blood pressure management for an acute dissection is a high priority with a goal of decreasing the systolic blood pressure (SBP) and force of contraction.

In the acute phase, this is accomplished by using an intravenous beta blocker, such as Esmolol or Labetalol, which are both negative inotropes. It is often used in conjunction with Nitroprusside or Nicardipine for successful reduction of SBP. Beta blockers have also been shown to reduce the risk of subsequent aneurysmal disease, therefore is it important to transition to oral beta blockers and possibly ACE inhibitors to manage the blood pressure. Intravenous calcium channel blockers like Diltiazem, have not proven more efficacious or effective over Esmolol in the acute phase.

70. D. Heart block. Heart block is a potential complication to anticipate after mitral or aortic valve replacement. This is related to disturbances to the Bundle of His. Anticipating heart blocks as a known complication includes being prepared to pace. Conduction disturbances can occur upwards of 15% of patients with MVRs, but are usually transient requiring short term, temporary pacing with only 1 - 3% requiring a permanent pacemaker.

71. D. Increase the Dobutamine infusion to 5 mcg/kg/min and reassess the hemodynamics in 15 minutes. The patient needs additional positive inotropic support to increase contractility and improve forward flow. The patient's filling pressures are adequate and would not benefit from diuretics or a fluid bolus. If the patient does not improve with an increase in Dobutamine, mechanical support like the IABP or Impella may be indicated.

72. B. Plays the organ at church every Sunday. Patients who work with their hands have an increased risk of debilitation from use of radial artery grafts for CABG. The patient's future of playing the organ may be jeopardized with radial grafting. In this case the risk vs. benefit of using the radial artery as a graft should be considered.

73. D. Synchronized cardioversion. Following the ACLS algorithm, the patient is unstable with signs of impaired perfusion including lightheadedness and sweaty with hypotension and a rapid irregular heart rate. Synchronized cardioversion is the appropriate immediate treatment. Amiodarone IV bolus may be considered if the patient was clinically stable. Termination of Atrial Fibrillation as quickly as possible post operatively is often the goal.

Note from Nicole—now let's get real...we'd likely try Amio or rate control before cardioversion despite the BP. For the exam (this one or ACLS), if the patient is in an unstable tachycardia that isn't sinus in nature, choose synchronized cardioversion. Real life might be different!

74. B. Prepare to administer Amiodarone 150 mg IV over 10 minutes. Given the relative stability of the patient, there is no need for synchronized cardioversion. The patient has converted into a stable Atrial Fibrillation. Cardizem (diltiazem) would not be the best option due to the potential of reduction in blood pressure. Adenosine is usually reserved for regular, narrow complex SVT rhythms. Amiodarone has the ability to slow the rate & convert the rhythm without causing hypotension. However, as you know Amiodarone has a very long half-life and a long list of side effects!

75. C. Respiratory acidosis. The pH is < 7.35 and $PaCO_2$ is > 45 mm Hg, both leaning toward acidosis. Without a change in the HCO_3 level, there is no evidence of compensation. This is likely an acute condition.

76. C. Initiate atrial pacing at rate of 80 beats/min. Utilizing temporary pacing to increase the heart rate to then increase the cardiac output should be the first intervention. Atrial pacing is preferred since the patient is in a sinus rhythm.

The patient's hemodynamics display adequate filling pressures and systemic vascular resistance, so giving additional fluid is not warranted at this time. The left and right stroke work index are not indicating that assistance is needed with contractility. Normal RVSWI is 5 - 10 g/m²/beat and normal LVSWI is 50 - 62 g/m²/beat. Therefore, initiating Dobutamine, in the setting of hypotension, with a normal systemic vascular resistance and stroke work index, may decrease SVR, worsening hypotension, and increase the risk of tachyarrhythmias.

Initiating Phenylephrine is not indicated in the setting of a normal SVR and may decrease the heart rate further, worsening cardiac output.

77. A. Notify the provider and prepare for pericardiocentesis. The patient is exhibiting classic signs of cardiac tamponade. Elevated right heart pressures with JVD, narrow pulse pressure, reduced mediastinal tube output and hypotension are signs of an emergency postoperative from cardiac tamponade. The provider should be notified immediately and preparations should be made for pericardiocentesis.

78. D. Decrease the set respiratory rate and tidal volume on the ventilator. The initial goal of acid-base balance is to achieve homeostasis by normalizing the pH with an attempt to compensate for the metabolic alkalosis. To compensate for a metabolic alkalosis, CO_2 must be retained. Decreasing the minute ventilation (rate and volume) will support increase in CO_2 retention. Fluid will not correct the metabolic imbalance of a significant base excess and there is no data to support the immediate incorporation of CRRT in the medical plan of care.

79. D. Volume resuscitation and vasopressors to maintain the MAP. Prolonged cardiopulmonary bypass time activates the inflammatory response. Histamine release causes significant vasodilation. Volume resuscitation and vasoconstrictors are important to promote venous return to the right side of the heart to improve preload and end-organ perfusion. The patient's SVR (afterload) should be monitored closely. Low SVR = vasodilation.

80. C. Worsening pulmonary hypertension. The indications for surgery in a patient with mitral stenosis include worsening pulmonary hypertension, NYHA class III or IV, infective endocarditis, systemic embolization and mitral valve area < 1.0 cm.

81. C. "This will eventually stop my irregular heart rhythm. Scar tissue does not conduct electrical signals." The MAZE procedure creates non-conductive scar tissue as incisions made in the heart muscle heals. Non-conducting scar tissue develops, creating a "maze" which disrupts the aberrant electrical signal. The procedure is often performed minimally invasive. The risk of blood clots exists and preventing thrombus formation will be a priority post-op.

82. A. Continue to monitor the patient and ensure proper timing of the IABP. Given the change in the patient's rhythm, hemodynamic stability is assessed by the augmented MAP on the balloon pump. Modern counterpulsation devices are able to switch from ECG to arterial BP triggering if needed to optimize timing of the IABP. Given the blood pressure is stable with a heart rate in the 80s, continue the counterpulsation therapy and monitor the patient. The nurse should report the rhythm change to the provider for consideration of rate or rhythm control.

83. B. Atrial fibrillation refractory to medication. The MAZE procedure creates non-conductive scar tissue as intentionally placed incisions in the heart muscle heals. The procedure is done to correct electrical and conduction problems refractory to traditional therapies such as medication and ablation. It is not a surgical procedure that will correct structural issues such as valve issues and septal wall defects.

84. D. Scratchy sound like Velcro. The characteristics of a pericardial friction rub resembles a scratchy sound like Velcro. It is constant rather than intermittent. A low rough rumbling sound is produced by stenotic murmurs. A high-pitched blowing sound may be heard with regurgitation murmurs.

85. A. Negative Allen's test on the left extremity. The Allen's Test assesses for insufficient blood flow to the hand from the ulnar artery. A negative Allen's test indicates the ability of the ulnar artery to perfuse the extremity is insufficient. The left radial artery should not be utilized for arterial puncture or grafting in this case.

86. C. Adenosine. Adenosine is the drug of choice in acute paroxysmal supraventricular tachycardia, if unresponsive to vagal maneuvers. If there is no response, consider using a beta blocker like metoprolol or esmolol or a calcium channel blocker like diltiazem (Cardizem) or verapamil. Synchronized cardioversion may be considered if the patient is unstable with signs of hypotension, cardiogenic shock, angina or CHF.

87. C. "I have been checking my blood glucose and using more insulin than I normally do." Surgery creates a stress response, which can increase blood glucose levels. However, uncontrolled blood glucose can result in delayed wound healing and result in increased risk for sternal wound infections. Walking and losing weight are expected goals post cardiac surgery. The patient is not taking warfarin, so eating spinach will not affect the patient's medication regimen.

88. A. Immediate surgery for repair. The dissection described is a Type A dissection. A Type A dissection is located on the ascending aort extending from the aortic valve. The extent of dissection can vary, but generally requires immediate surgical repair. Type B dissections, or aortic dissections of the descending aorta can be considered for initial medical management with anti-hypertensives and may require surgery or stenting long term.

89. C. Perform the CIWA assessment and notify the provider. The patient is likely undergoing alcohol withdrawal. The severity of symptoms should be assessed by a reliable and valid assessment tool such as Clinical Institute Withdrawal Assessment (CIWA). The severity of withdrawal and symptoms will determine the pharmacologic intervention. If the patient is indeed going through alcohol withdrawal, benzodiazepine administration would be indicated. Protocols vary and other medications such as Dexmedetomidine (Precedex) or Librium may be used. Placement of an advanced airway is only indicated if the patient cannot maintain their airway.

90. B. "Cross clamping the aorta can impact perfusion to the spinal cord." Cross clamping the aorta increases the risk of paralysis due to decreased perfusion to the spinal cord. A lumbar drain is placed to minimize compression of the spinal cord with CSF post-operatively. Frequent assessments of lower extremity movement and sensation should be a priority post operatively.

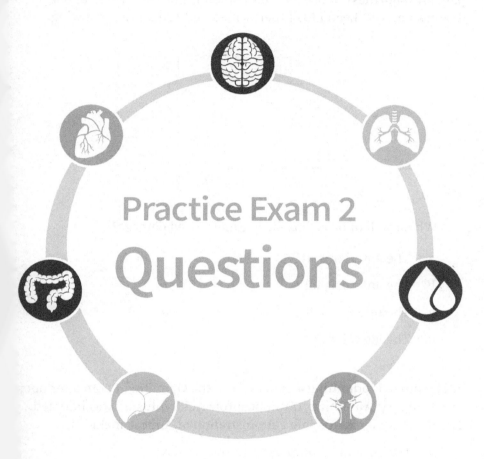

Practice Exam 2
Questions

Practice Exam 2

1. A 73-year-old male presents to the hospital with a complaint of chest pain and shortness of breath. The Troponin-I level is elevated, but decreasing. A 12-Lead ECG is performed and reveals the following:

Which wall of heart has likely experienced damage?

    a.   The anterior wall

    b.   The anteroseptal wall

    c.   The inferior wall

    d.   The lateral wall

2. The nurse is admitting a patient from the Operating Room after oper heart surgery. An Amicar (Aminocaproic Acid) infusion was initiated. The nurse understands safe administration of Amicar includes:

    a.   Dosing a maximum of 30 grams per day.

    b.   Continue administration despite the cessation of bleeding.

    c.   It does not impact fibrinolysis.

    d.   It has a half-life > 12 hours.

3. While precepting a student nurse, you are explaining the benefit of using intra-aortic balloon counterpulsation in the setting of cardiogenic shock post cardiac surgery. Which of the following would be an accurate description of this therapy?

    a.   The balloon inflates during systole to reduce afterload and the pressure the left ventricle must pump against

    b.   The balloon inflates during diastole to improve coronary, cerebral and peripheral blood flow

    c.   The balloon deflates during diastole to increase cardiac output, ejection fraction and forward flow

    d.   The balloon inflates during systole to push blood retrograde towards arch and forward flow toward the periphery

4. A Rapid Response was activated on the surgical floor for a 25-year old patient post-op day 5 after heart transplant. On assessment the patient is diaphoretic, nauseated and lightheaded.

Vital signs on arrival:

HR 40 bpm

BP 76/40 (52) mm Hg

RR 24

What is the priority action by the nurse?

    a.   Administer 1 mg Atropine IV

    b.   Begin Epinephrine (Adrenaline) infusion

    c.   Connect epicardial pacing wires and begin pacing

    d.   Administer 1 liter lactated ringers bolus

5. A nurse is caring for a patient who is post-operative from an aortic and mitral valve replacement.

Current vital signs and hemodynamics:

HR: 102 bpm

BP: 80/42 (55) via arterial line

SpO_2: 99% on 30% FiO_2

CO: 4.8 L/min

CI: 2.2 L/min/m^2

CVP: 12 mm Hg

PAP: 32/16 mm Hg

PAOP: 14 mm Hg

SvO_2 64%

SV: 62 ml/beat

SVR: 478 dynes/sec/cm^{-5}

Which of the following medications should be initiated?

a.   Dobutamine infusion

b.   Nitroglycerin infusion

c.   Milrinone infusion

d.   Phenylephrine infusion

6. A 39-year-old male patient is 10 days postoperative from a 3-vessel CABG. The patient progressed well postoperatively. However, during the last three days, oxygen requirements have increased. A chest radiograph demonstrates increased consolidation in the right lower lung with bilateral pulmonary infiltrates. Despite antibiotics, the patient is now intubated and a PA catheter was placed.

ABG results:

pH 7.20

$PaCO_2$ 63

PaO_2 68

HCO_3 28

Vent settings:

AMV mode

Vt 560

Set rate 18

PEEP +12

FiO_2 100%

Hemodynamics:

CO: 5.6 L/min	PAOP: 8 mm Hg
CI: 2.8 L/min/m²	SvO₂ 58%
CVP: 14 mm Hg	SV: 86 ml/beat
PAP: 32/16 mm Hg	SVR: 662 dynes/sec/cm⁻⁵

Based on the clinical values, the patient is demonstrating signs of:

a. Atelectasis

b. Hemothorax

c. Acute Respiratory Distress Syndrome

d. Pulmonary Hypertension

7. A patient arrives to the ICU after a pericardial window following blunt cardiac trauma.

Patient data on arrival:	**Patient data 1 hour later:**
HR 102	HR 130
BP 102/56 (71) mm H	BP 80/70 (73) mm Hg
CVP 5 mm Hg	CVP 16 mm Hg
Chest tube output 75 ml	Chest tube output 0 ml

Based on the clinical picture and hemodynamics, which complication should the nurse suspect?

a. Pleural effusion

b. Pulmonary embolism

c. Pulsus paradoxus

d. Cardiac tamponade

8. A 68-year-old female who had a CABG 7 days prior is readmitted to the ICU from the Emergency Department with shortness of breath. The provider placed a PA catheter to assess hemodynamics and pulmonary pressures to guide therapy.

HR 95 bpm

BP 114/68

C.O. 3.1 L/min

C.I. 1.6 L/min/m²

PA 48/26 mm Hg

PAOP 10 mm Hg

CVP 8 mm Hg

SvO₂ 48%

An arterial blood gas was obtained and reveals the following:

pH 7.26

$PaCO_2$ 69

PaO_2 52

HCO_3 29

The patient is electively intubated & mechanically ventilated on AMV mode, rate 18, 100% FiO_2, +15 PEEP.

Which of the following treatments is most evidence-based to improve the refractory hypoxemia in the settings of ARDS?

a. Nebulized Albuterol

b. Nebulized Epoprostenol (Flolan)

c. IV steroids

d. Prone positioning

9. A 60-year-old male patient arrives to the ICU after a coronary artery bypass graft surgery (CABG). On assessment the heart tones are muffled and jugular venous distension is visible. Which clinical data supports the nurse's suspicion of cardiac tamponade?

a. BP 88/70 (76) and CVP 18 mm Hg

b. BP 160/40 (80) and CVP 4 mm Hg

c. HR 40 and CVP 12 mm Hg

d. HR 140 and BP 158/44 (82)

10. Your patient is post-operative day 1 after a 2-vessel CABG. The patient is receiving Epinephrine, Insulin, D5NS and Amiodarone infusions. The hemodynamics are improving and Epinephrine has been weaned off. What other infusion do you anticipate weaning down because of the decreased Epinephrine needs?

   a. Insulin

   b. D5NS

   c. Amiodarone

   d. No changes are necessary

11. You are caring for a patient with an acute arterial occlusion in left lower extremity. Which of the following clinical findings are associated with this diagnosis?

   a. Pallor, bounding pulse, delayed capillary refill, pain

   b. Pain, pulseless, pallor, poor skin turgor

   c. Polar, pulseless, pallor, pain

   d. Pain, paresthesia, bounding pulse, polar

12. Which of the following scenarios would necessitate a resternotomy procedure at the bedside following an aortic valve replacement?

   a. Hemodynamic instability caused by cardiac tamponade

   b. Chest tube output of 150 ml/hour for 2 hours

   c. ST elevation on the 12 lead ECG

   d. Sustained ventricular tachycardia

13. The following patient data is noted 2 hours after the patient arrives to the ICU post cardiac surgery:

HR 122

BP 74/68 (70)

CVP 22 mm Hg

PAP 48/22 mm Hg

Chest tube output: none

The nurse assesses muffled heart tones, weak thready pulses and significant jugular venous distension. Which emergent intervention should the nurse anticipate?

a.   Chest tube placement

b.   TTE

c.   Bedside re-sternotomy

d.   Intra-aortic balloon pump placement

14. A 38-year-old male who is post-operative cardiac bypass surgery demonstrates the following vital signs:

HR 98 bpm

BP 95/53 (67) mm Hg via arterial line

CVP 10 mm Hg

PA 25/16 mm Hg

PAOP 16 mm Hg

C.O. 3.2 L/min

C.I 1.8 L/min/m^2

SVR 1830 dynes/sec/cm^{-5}

Based on the hemodynamic profile, which of the following medications should be administered?

a.   1 liter Lactated Ringers IV bolus

b.   Epinephrine infusion

c.   Dopamine infusion

d.   Dobutamine infusion

15. On arrival to the ICU following a right lower lobectomy for lung cancer, the patient has two pleural chest tubes to -20 cm wall suction. Tidaling is visible in both water seal chambers. The chest tube output is as follows:

Chest tube #1 - 125 ml sanguineous drainage

Chest tube #2 - 150 ml sanguineous drainage

What is the appropriate next action by the nurse?

a.   Document the findings and continue to monitor

b.   Strip the chest tube tubing

c.   Turn off the suction and place the chest tubes to water seal

d.   Slide the clamp closed on the drainage tubing

16. A patient is admitted to the ICU post LVAD implantation. The patient is mechanically ventilated on Assist Control.

The patient's vital signs are as follows:

HR 95 bpm	PAP 37/24 mm Hg
MAP 62 mm Hg	PAOP 14 mm Hg
Cardiac Index 1.9 L/min/m^2	SvO$_2$ 52%
CVP 20 mm Hg	

The patient is on Milrinone at 1.0 mcg/kg/min and Epinephrine at 0.75 mcg/kg/min. Which of the following should be considered?

a.   Inhaled nitric oxide

b.   Beta blockers

c.   Wean the Milrinone infusion

d.   Administer a Phenylephrine infusion

17. To reduce spinal cord ischemia in the setting of descending aorta aneurysm, which of the following interventions should be done?

a.   Maintain MAP < 80 mm Hg

b.   Place the patient in the reverse Trendelenburg position

c.   Initiate a Norepinephrine infusion to keep the MAP > 65 mm Hg

d.   Open the lumbar drain to decrease cerebral spinal pressure

18. A patient in the ICU one hour post cardiac surgery, has a sudden output of 500 ml of sanguineous drainage from the mediastinal chest tubes. A massive transfusion protocol is initiated, including packed red blood cells (PRBCs), fresh frozen plasma (FFP) and platelets. Which electrolyte should the nurse anticipate replacing?

a.   Calcium

b.   Potassium

c.   Magnesium

d.   Phosphorus

19. A nurse receives a 48-year-old male admitted with a STEMI secondary to left anterior descending (LAD) occlusion. The 12 lead ECG reveals ST elevation in leads V1 – V4 and a new harsh holosystolic murmur is auscultated. Which of the following complications is suspected to cause the hypotension and murmur?

    a. Reperfusion injury

    b. Ventricular aneurysm

    c. Septal rupture

    d. Cardiomyopathy

20. A patient with a left ventricular assist device (LVAD) presents to the Emergency Department with an acute onset of congestive heart failure symptoms. Pump thrombosis is suspected. Clinical findings to support this diagnosis include which of the following?

    a. Elevated hematocrit

    b. Decrease in left ventricular diastolic volume

    c. Decreased serum lactate dehydrogenase (LDH)

    d. Hemoglobinuria

21. The nurse is called to the bedside of a patient post-op day 3 after a thoracotomy whose mobility has been limited by pain. The patient feels short of breath with diminished lung sounds to the right side.

Patient data:

HR 110

BP 122/70 (87) mm Hg

RR 40

SpO_2 88% on 5 L NC

Which order should the nurse anticipate as a priority?

a. BiPAP 50% FiO_2

b. Chest x-ray STAT

c. Arterial blood gas (ABG)

d. Chest percussion every 2 hours

22. Which of the following 12 lead ECG findings interfere with detecting ischemia?

a. First degree AV conduction delay

b. Left bundle branch block

c. Atrial paced rhythm

d. Right ventricular hypertrophy

23. An 83-year-old female is post-operative from an uncomplicated trans-apical TAVR. The most likely complication from this procedure is:

a. Anemia

b. Bleeding

c. Delirium

d. Ventricular arrhythmias

24. A 58-year-old male who experienced a STEMI, is now 3 days post-operative from a 3-vessel CABG. Prior to surgery the patient was anticoagulated with Heparin in the Cath lab. The RN notes the patient developing petechiae over the past two days. Today, the patient's toes are purple with pulses detected only with Doppler. The RN should anticipate which of the following interventions?

a.   Stop the Heparin infusion, HIT is suspected

b.   Hold groin pressure, a retroperitoneal bleed is suspected

c.   Perform a neurological exam, a stroke is suspected

d.   Send a stat coagulation panel, the patient is likely bleeding

25. A 50-year-old patient with a history of Stage 3 COPD is extubated 3 hours post CABG. A post extubation arterial blood gas (ABG) is sent.

The patient's vital signs are as follows:

HR 68

BP 110/58 (75) mm Hg

RR 22

T 36.8° C

SpO_2 93% on room air

Considering the patient's chronic lung disease, which ABG would the nurse anticipate?

	pH	$PaCO_2$	PaO_2	HCO_3
a.	7.55	30	80	30
b.	7.20	70	60	36
c.	7.39	48	65	28
d.	7.40	42	80	26

26. A 100 kg male remains on mechanical ventilation following a 3 vessel CABG. A video assisted thorascopic surgery (VATS) was performed due to increased oxygen needs.

Arterial blood gas results:	Vent settings:
pH 7.48	Vt 800 ml (8 mL/kg)
$PaCO_2$ 32	AMV mode
PaO_2 85	Set rate 16
HCO_3 25	60% FiO_2
	+ 8 PEEP

A bedside echocardiogram was performed and did not reveal abnormalities. A chest radiograph shows worsening bilateral opacities. The next most appropriate evidenced based treatment is:

a. Increase the FiO_2 to 100%

b. Monitor the patient and repeat an ABG and CXR in 2 hours

c. Decrease the tidal volume to 6 ml/kg

d. Increase the tidal volume to 8.5 ml/kg

27. The nurse receives an order for an atrial electrocardiogram for a post-operative patient with new onset supraventricular tachycardia. To perform the atrial electrocardiogram, the nurse:

a. Connects the atrial pacing wire to the RA lead

b. Connects the atrial pacing wire to the V lead

c. Connects the ventricular pacing wire to the V lead

d. Connects the ventricular pacing wire to the LA lead

28. A 47-year-old female patient is in the immediate post-operative phase after a mitral valve repair and aortic valve replacement. While receiving the patient from OR, the RN notes Ventricular Fibrillation on

the transport monitor. What should be the first intervention & highest priority to treat this lethal arrhythmia?

a. Synchronized Cardioversion

b. Defibrillation with 200 joules

c. Initiate Transcutaneous Pacing

d. Amiodarone 300 mg followed by an infusion

29. Which of the following patients is at highest risk for developing an ischemic stroke after a 3-vessel CABG?

a. 45-year-old male who smokes

b. 82-year-old female with emphysema

c. 72-year-old male with diabetes

d. 50-year-old female with cirrhosis

30. You are caring for a patient status post mechanical mitral valve replacement, who is now post-op day 2. During morning multidisciplinary rounds, it was identified that the platelet count dropped from 152,000 mm³ to 48,000 mm³ since admission, but the PT/INR is normal. Which of the following orders do you anticipate?

a. Discontinue any form of Heparin and start warfarin

b. Discontinue warfarin and start unfractionated Heparin

c. Discontinue warfarin and give Fresh Frozen Plasma (FFP)

d. Discontinue any form of Heparin and start Argatroban

31. A 68-year-old patient with COPD has developed ARDS following cardiac surgery requiring increased PEEP while intubated. The nurse understands which assessment findings would be seen with the complication of pneumomediastinum?

   a.   Back pain and muffled heart tones

   b.   Decreased lung sounds and stridor

   c.   Pulsus paradoxus and decreased chest tube drainage

   d.   Crepitus along the sternal border and distant heart tones

32. A 64-year-old male patient is s/p thoracic aortic aneurysm repair with endograft. The arterial line is in the right radial artery and reads 120/80 (93) mm Hg. The RN notes the left arm is dusky in comparison and capillary refill is > 3 seconds. The pulse is weak and barely audible by Doppler. The RN should:

   a.   Assess the blood pressure in the left arm

   b.   Assess bilateral lower extremity pulses

   c.   Monitor urine output and send a stat BUN and creatinine

   d.   Send stat coagulation labs

33. A patient with new onset Atrial Fibrillation with a ventricular rate of 155 bpm after mitral valve replacement (MVR) is prescribed Amiodarone (Cordarone) IV bolus over 10 minutes followed by an infusion. Which changes in the patient's rhythm should the nurse anticipate with administration of Amiodarone (Cordarone)?

   a.   A prolonged pause with resumption of normal sinus rhythm

   b.   A control of the Atrial Fibrillation with a ventricular rate below 100 beats per minute with a shortened QT interval

   c.   Conversion of the rhythm to sinus and slowing of the ventricular response

   d.   A delay in conduction at the AV junction

34. When caring for a patient with epicardial pacing wires, what is the optimal way to secure the wires when not in use?

    a.   Bunch them all together and wind tape around them to secure them.

    b.   Leave them open to air and without dressings.

    c.   Insulate the atrial wires separate from the ventricular wires to prevent cross-communication.

    d.   Wrap them around the chest tubes.

35. Which of the following ICU patients should be placed on GI prophylaxis?

    a.   56-year-old with pneumonia on antibiotics

    b.   68-year-old ICU day 4 post coronary artery bypass

    c.   35-year-old admitted to the ICU with heart failure

    d.   60-year-old with liver failure and an initial INR of 2.5

36. When educating your patient and their family regarding management of infective endocarditis, which of the following interventions are expected?

    a. Anticoagulation

    b. Oral antibiotic therapy for 2 weeks

    c. IV antibiotic therapy for 6 weeks

    d. Valve repair

37. Your patient returns from the OR after a mitral valve replacement &

has ventricular epicardial wires in place.

Hemodynamics:

HR: 50 bpm

BP: 70/32 (45)

CO: 4.5 L/min

CI: 2.1 L/min/m²

SV: 52 ml/beat

CVP: 8 mm Hg

PAOP: 12 mm Hg

SVR: 854 dynes/sec/cm⁻⁵

What should be the initial action & priority?

   a.   Discuss an immediate return to the OR with the cardiac surgeon.

   b.   Connect the epicardial wires to the pacemaker and emergently VVI pace.

   c.   Initiate an Epinephrine infusion.

   d.   Infuse a crystalloid bolus.

38. The RN is assessing a patient post mitral valve repair. When evaluating the hemodynamics, the nurse notes cyclical changes in the arterial pressure line. The arterial blood pressure waveform is narrow and lower when the patient inhales compared to when they exhale. This variation in the arterial line pressures describes which of the following?

   a.   Pulsus Alternans

   b.   Pulsus Bigeminis

   c.   Pulsus Variation

   d.   Pulsus Paradoxus

39. A patient is admitted to the ICU following a mitral valve

replacement (MVR). A Pulmonary Artery catheter is in place.

The patient's vital signs are as follows:

HR 100 bpm

BP 86/42 (57) mm Hg

CVP 8 mm Hg

PAP 38/18 (25) mm Hg

PAOP 16 mm Hg

CI 1.9 L/min/m²

SVR 1850 dynes/sec/cm⁻⁵

Based on the hemodynamic profile, which order should the nurse anticipate?

a. Begin a Vasopressin infusion

b. Begin a Dobutamine infusion

c. Begin a Norepinephrine infusion

d. Administer a Lactated Ringers fluid bolus

40. Upon reading the patient's history, the RN discovers they have von Willebrand disease and allergies to fish. Which of the following medications should you be prepared to administer to help promote hemostasis, in the setting of postoperative bleeding?

a. Prothrombin Complex Concentrate (Kcentra®)

b. Desmopressin acetate (DDAVP)

c. Protamine sulfate

d. Phentolamine mesylate (Regitine)

41. A patient arrives to the ICU immediately following a mitral valve

replacement (MVR).

Vital signs are as follows:

HR 80 bpm

BP 112/42 (65) mm Hg

CVP 14 mm Hg

PAP 46/18 (27) mm Hg

CI 1.8 L/min/m²

SVR 1780 dynes/sec/cm⁻⁵

SvO₂ 52%

Chest tube output 125 ml

Urine output 50 ml

Dobutamine is ordered to infuse at 2.5 mcg/kg/min. Which assessment findings would the nurse anticipate after the Dobutamine administration?

a.   An increase in the SvO_2

b.   An increase in the SVR

c.   A decrease in urine output

d.   An decrease in the cardiac index

42. A patient is experiencing post-operative bleeding after a 3 vesse CABG. The mediastinal chest tube output has been 100 - 150 mL/hou and is sanguineous. The patient's coagulation panel reveals the following

Hgb 8.3 g/dL

Hct 25%

PTT 36 seconds

PT/INR 13.9/1.1 seconds

Platelet 152 thousand/uL

Fibrinogen 80 mg/dL

The RN should anticipate which of the following?

a.   Packed Red Blood Cells

b.   Platelets

c.   Fresh Frozen Plasma

d.   Cryoprecipitate

43. A patient post mitral valve replacement (MVR) is ordered to start a Milrinone (Primacor) infusion. Which lab values are a priority for the nurse to monitor?

    a. Serum electrolytes

    b. Blood glucose

    c. Hematocrit

    d. Lactate

44. The nurse is caring for a patient with a temporary transvenous pacemaker set to a backup ventricular rate of 55 bpm. The monitor shows a pacing spike that is not immediately followed by a QRS complex. The patient is unstable with a blood pressure of 80/42 (55) mm Hg and is difficult to arouse.

    What should be the initial action?

    a. Increase the energy (mA)

    b. Administer Atropine 0.5 mg IV

    c. Increase the sensitivity setting

    d. Administer Lactated Ringers 500 ml IV

45. Cyanosis in adults with congenital heart defects is caused by left to right shunting of blood. The most common cause of cyanosis in an adult with a congenital heart defect is:

    a. Eisenmenger Syndrome

    b. Pulmonary hypertension

    c. Anemia

    d. Tetralogy of Fallot

46. You are caring for a 56-year-old male status post anterior wall MI and 3-vessel CABG with bypass grafts to the left anterior descending (LAD), circumflex (CX), and right coronary artery (RCA). The most recent vital signs reveal HR 115, BP 86/70 (66), RR 22, and SpO$_2$ 94% on 4 liters oxygen per nasal cannula.

> The patient has a Pulmonary Artery catheter in place. The most recent hemodynamic calculations reveal:
>
> Cardiac index (CI) 1.7 L/min/m^2
>
> Stroke volume index (SVI) 24 ml/beat/m^2
>
> Left ventricular work index (LVSWI) 14 g/m^2/beat
>
> Right ventricular stroke work index (RVSWI) 3 g/m^2/beat
>
> SVR 2100 dynes/sec/cm^{-5}
>
> SvO$_2$ 52%
>
> Which of the following medications are a priority to improve perfusion and oxygen delivery?
>
> a.   Dobutamine
>
> b.   Phenylephrine
>
> c.   Vasopressin
>
> d.   Norepinephrine

47. A patient who experienced a prolonged bypass time in the OR is now confused and agitated. The provider orders haloperidol (Haldol) for the patient. What should the nurse be concerned with in regard to the administration of Haldol?

    a.   Prolonged QT interval

    b.   Atrial fibrillation

    c.   Respiratory failure

    d.   Acute Kidney Injury

48. A patient arrives to the ICU following surgical aortic valve replacement for aortic regurgitation. Which pharmacologic intervention should the nurse anticipate immediately postoperative?

    a. Norepinephrine (Levophed)

    b. Milrinone (Primacor)

    c. Vasopressin (Pitressin)

    d. Losartan (Cozaar)

49. A 19-year-old male presents to the Emergency Department for shortness of breath. The patient states he was born in a small village in Somalia. He has always had shortness of breath and never been able to run or walk up a flight of stairs without passing out.

Vital signs are as follows:

HR 122 bpm

BP 122/90 mm Hg

RR 30 bpm

SpO_2 84% on room air

Temp 37.5° C

The RN is assessing the patient and hears crackles in all lung fields. His CXR demonstrates pulmonary edema. A holosystolic murmur is ausalated on his left lower sternal border. Which of the following diagnosis is most likely causing his current state of health?

    a. Asthma

    b. Pulmonary Embolism

    c. Pneumonia

    d. Ventricular Septal Defect

50. A 48-year-old male s/p left lower lobectomy has recently had his chest tube placed to water seal. The patient becomes short of breath, tachypneic and has decreased oxygen saturation. Bubbling is noted in the water seal chamber. The first intervention by the nurse should be:

    a.   Obtain a stat portable chest radiograph

    b.   Obtain an arterial blood gas

    c.   Administer albuterol stat

    d.   Place the chest tube to suction

51. You are caring for a patient, status post anterior wall MI and 4-vessel coronary artery bypass grafting who has a Pulmonary Artery catheter in place. You suddenly notice large v waves on the pulmonary artery occlusion pressure (PAOP) waveform. Which of the following can cause large v waves on the PAOP waveform?

    a.   Decreased atrial filling

    b.   Tricuspid regurgitation

    c.   Acute mitral regurgitation

    d.   Right ventricular failure

52. The nurse is performing an initial assessment on a patient who is post-operative day 3 following cardiac surgery. The nurse notes the bilateral upper extremity movements are not equal and the right hand grasp is weaker than the left. The patient is having trouble reading the white board with noted double vision.

Vital signs are as follows:

HR 92 bpm

BP 130/72 (91) mm Hg

RR 18

SpO_2 98% on 2 L NC

Which order should the nurse anticipate?

a. Heparin infusion

b. STAT head CT Scan with NIH stroke scale assessment

c. Alteplase (Activase) IV bolus STAT

d. Neurologic assessments every hour

53. The nurse is caring for a patient who returned from an aortic valve replacement 45 minutes ago. Suddenly, the nurse notes shivering, heart rate increasing to 107 bpm from 70 bpm, and the SvO_2 decreased to 47%. Which of the following interventions should be anticipated?

a. Neuromuscular blockade

b. Meperidine (Demerol) 25 mg IV push

c. Increase the FiO_2

d. Buspirone 30 mg per gastric tube

54. A 62-year-old male is 4 hours post-operative from an aortic valve replacement due to aortic stenosis. The patient was extubated in the operating room. The patient is talking to his wife at the bedside. The wife pushes the call bell to tell the nurse the patient is having trouble finding his words and speech is slurred.

The RN should prioritize which of the following actions first?

a. Perform a stat capillary glucose

b. Perform a complete National Institute of Health (NIH) Stroke Scale assessment

c. Prepare to administer Naloxone

d. Prepare for a stat head CT scan

55. Post-operative orders for a patient s/p esophagectomy include maintaining the head of bed position at 30 degrees at all times. The rationale for positioning is:

   a. To promote chest tube drainage

   b. To prevent gastric aspiration into the lungs

   c. To prevent diaphragmatic hernia

   d. To offload pressure on the sacrum and prevent skin breakdown

56. The nurse is caring for a patient with a temporary transvenous pacemaker set to a backup ventricular rate of 55 bpm. The nurse notices while the patient is sleeping, they are more dependent on the pacemaker. However, the monitor showed a pacing spike that was not immediately followed by a QRS complex. The patient is hemodynamically stable.

   What should be the initial action?

   a. Perform an energy threshold to determine the proper energy (mA) setting

   b. Perform a sensitivity threshold to determine the proper sensitivity (mV) setting

   c. Decrease the sensitivity (mV) setting

   d. Administer 0.5 mg Atropine IV

57. An obese 52-year-old man with a history of Atrial Fibrillation is recovering from open-heart surgery for aortic valve replacement and 3-vessel CABG. To decrease the risk of developing postoperative Atrial Fibrillation, which of the following medications is most commonly administered for prophylaxis?

a.   Magnesium sulfate

b.   Diltiazem

d.   Aspirin

d.   Metoprolol

58. A patient arrives from the operating room with a temporary pacemaker generator connected to epicardial pacing wires. The bedside ECG rhythm shows atrial pacer spikes without subsequent atrial depolarization and P waves. Which action should the nurse prioritize?

a.   Increase the atrial mA

b.   Decrease the atrial sensitivity

c.   Order a STAT chest x-ray

d.   Obtain serum electrolytes

59. An appropriate antithrombotic medication regimen following a transcatheter aortic valve replacement (TAVR) for a patient without a contraindication to anticoagulation is:

a.   Aspirin 75 mg – 100 mg daily

b.   Clopidogrel (Plavix) 75 mg daily

c.   Aspirin 75 mg – 100 mg daily and Clopidogrel (Plavix) 75 mg daily

d.   Warfarin (Coumadin) for a target INR of 2 – 3

60. A 58-year-old male is admitted to CVICU 4 hours postoperative after 1-vessel CABG. He remains on an Insulin infusion, Norepinephrine and Dobutamine. His vital signs remain stable postoperatively. The patient continues to complain he is cold and sweaty, despite his PA catheter temperature reading of 37.3°C. The patient also states he is super sleepy" and "I feel nervous and shaky." The RN should anticipate which of the following?

   a.   A complete neurological examination

   b.   Explain to the patient this is normal postoperatively

   c.   Assess a blood glucose level

   d.   Increase the Dobutamine infusion

61. The nurse is caring for a patient after dual chamber permanent pacemaker placement. The settings on the pacemaker are such that the atria and ventricles are paced, sensing occurs in the atria and ventricles, and atrial sensing inhibits atrial pacing while ventricular sensing inhibits ventricular pacing. The nurse documents this pacing mode as:

   a.   DDI

   b.   VDD

   c.   DVI

   d.   DDD

62. While caring for a patient immediately upon return from the OR, the Respiratory Therapist is adjusting the ventilator settings to support the patient's needs. Upon increasing the PEEP, the patient's blood pressure drops. What is likely the cause of the hypotension?

   a.   The decrease in blood pressure and the increase in PEEP have no correlation

   b.   Negative pressure ventilation; whenever the patient exhales it creates a suction pressure to the chest, dropping the blood pressure

   c.   The patient is bleeding and needs immediate return to the OR for exploration

   d.   Positive pressure ventilation; when the patient inhales, the increased pressure creates added pressure on the thoracic cavity

63. A nurse is caring for a patient receiving intravenous Heparin due to a left ventricular thrombus and are concerned for Heparin Induced Thrombocytopenia (HIT). The RN calculates the patient's "4 T score" to be 6 (high probability of HIT). Which of the following actions would be most appropriate?

    a.   Stop the Heparin infusion and send labs to confirm HIT diagnosis.

    b.   Continue the Heparin infusion and labs to confirm HIT diagnosis.

    c.   Stop the Heparin infusion, start Bivalirudin and send labs to confirm HIT diagnosis.

    d.   Continue the Heparin infusion and do not send labs to confirm HIT diagnosis.

64. The nurse is caring for 74-year-old female 19 hours after a minimally invasive mitral valve replacement. The patient self-extubated 6 hours previously and her chest tubes stopped draining just prior to that. The RN observes she is currently anxious, tachypneic with nasal flaring and clavicular retractions has Pulsus paradoxus on the arterial line tracing, and a low voltage QRS with tachycardia on the bedside monitor with electrical alternans.

Vital signs:

HR 145 bpm

ABP 81/75 (58) mm Hg

SpO$_2$ 89% on 10 L high flow nasal cannula

Cardiac Index (CI) 1.7 L/min/m^2

Stroke Volume Index (SVI) 17 mL/beat/m^2

CVP 24 mm Hg

PAP 55/25 mm Hg

PAOP 26 mm Hg

SVR 2350 dyne/sec/cm^{-5}

Right Ventricular Stroke Work Index (RVSWI) 1.3 g/m^2/beat

Left Ventricular Stroke Work Index (LVSWI) 11 g/m^2/beat

The patient is currently on Epinephrine @ 0.5 mcg/kg/min, Norepinephrine @ 1 mcg/kg/min, Vasopressin @ 0.4 units/min and Dobutamine @ 5 mcg/kg/min.

Which of the following is the appropriate intervention?

a. Increase the Epinephrine infusion

b. Prepare for pericardiocentesis and/or re-sternotomy

c. Increase the Vasopressin infusion

d. Increase the Dobutamine infusion

65. A patient in the ICU post heart transplantation is at risk for developing right sided heart failure. The nurse understands this is related to:

a. Increased pulmonary vascular resistance (PVR)

b. Historical development of chronic kidney disease

c. Acute organ rejection

d. Excessive diuretic use without electrolyte replacement

66. A 68-year-old male is admitted to the ICU s/p thoracic endovascular aortic aneurysm repair with a lumbar drain in place. Orders are received to level the transducer to the patient's iliac crest and place the drip chamber to maintain a CSF pressure ≤ 13 mm Hg. The patient's CSF pressure is now reading 20 mm Hg. An appropriate intervention would be to:

a. Raise the device 20 cm H_2O and keep open to drain

b. Raise the device to 15 cm H_2O and keep open to drain

c. Lower the device to 10 cm H_2O and clamp

d. Lower the device to 10 cm H_2O and keep open to drain

67. Post-operative incision care strategies to minimize the risk of surgical site infection includes:

    a. Glycemic control, body shaving, impermeable dressings left in place for 1 week

    b. Glycemic control, chlorhexidine bathing, dry sterile dressing

    c. Hydrogen peroxide daily to incision, glycemic control, chlorhexidine bathing

    d. Chlorhexidine bathing, antibiotic ointment to surgical incision, body hair shaving

68. The RN is caring for an 88-year-old female 12 hours post open-heart surgery for coronary artery bypass grafting x 5 and redo aortic valve replacement. Upon dangling for the first time, she has complaints of dizziness, becomes hypotensive and tachycardic. The RN notices an additional 275 ml of dark red blood in the mediastinal chest tubes. After notifying the surgeon, which of the following interventions should be anticipated?

    a. Suction the chest tubes

    b. Give back blood in chest tubes via auto-transfusion

    c. Strip the chest tubes

    d. Draw stat labs to assess coagulation studies and complete blood count

69. The nurse is receiving report from the Operating Room in the care of a patient coming off bypass for coronary artery bypass grafting (CABG). The nurse is informed there was a suspected Protamine reaction with a significant drop in blood pressure and systemic vascular resistance. The nurse anticipates which medication was administered in the operating room in response to the possible reaction?

    a.   Methylene blue IV infusion

    b.   Fresh frozen plasma (FFP) 2 units STAT

    c.   Heparin 10,000 units IV

    d.   Vitamin K (Phytonadione) 10 mg IV infusion

70. The patient is doing well 4 hours post-op, but the RN has noticed the chest tube output has suddenly ceased. Twenty minutes later the patient is becoming tachycardic, hypotensive and the pulmonary artery and central venous pressures are equalizing. The nurse gets an immediate chest radiograph and notes the mediastinum is wider than the initial x-ray. What should the nurse suspect based on these findings?

    a.   Nothing, these are normal postoperative signs and symptoms

    b.   The PA catheter must be dislodged; call the provider to reposition the catheter

    c.   Cardiac tamponade; call the provider immediately and prepare to suction the chest tubes & possible re-sternotomy

    d.   Pneumonia; infiltrates are likely the cause of the widened mediastinum

71. Which of the following class of medications has demonstrated reduced risk of death, recurrent MI, stroke, and future need for revascularization with acute coronary syndrome (ACS)?

    a.   Statins

    b.   Nitrates

    c. P_2Y_{12} inhibitors

    d.   Glycoprotein IIb/IIIa inhibitors

72. The nurse is caring for a patient 24 hours post aortic valve replacement. The patient asks why the ECG cables can't be taken off yet. Which response by the nurse is most appropriate?

    a. "The provider would like to see your heart rhythm for a few days."

    b. "You're doing fine, I'm sure it will be discontinued today."

    c. "There is a risk of changes to your heart rhythm after surgery and it is important to monitor."

    d. "There is a risk your heart could stop and I need to be watching it continuously."

73. A nurse is mentoring a new nurse caring for a patient receiving counter-pulsation therapy with an intra-aortic balloon pump (IABP). In review of the IABP waveform, which of the following is the best assessment of improved coronary blood flow?

    a. Unassisted systole

    b. Augmented diasolic pressure

    c. Aortic end-diastolic pressure

    d. Assisted systole

74. An 83-year-old male is admitted to the Cardiothoracic ICU post transcatheter aortic valve replacement (TAVR) and is requiring transvenous VVI pacing post procedure. The most likely cause for heart block after this procedure is:

    a. Advancement of the guidewire prior to deployment

    b. Long term beta blockade pre-procedure

    c. Chronic conduction system disease

    d. Valve expansion after deployment

75. An 82-year-old female is now post-operative day 14 after a 4-vessel CABG. The patient was a DNR at her assisted living facility, but her family convinced her that she needed the surgery so that she could "live chest pain free." The patient was extubated post-operatively per protocol. She initially was compliant in the plan of care, but each day she has progressively become more withdrawn and lethargic and is not eating. Two days ago during rounds, she developed respiratory distress and was re-intubated per her family's wishes. The RN should:

   a. Continue to follow the family's wishes

   b. Request a patient care conference to discuss the patient's wishes

   c. Respect the patient's DNR wishes and extubate the patient

   d. Consult a legal guardian outside the hospital

76. A patient just arrived from the OR post 5-vessel CABG. The patient has one pleural and two mediastinal chest tubes in place. The RN notices air bubbles in the water seal chamber in the chest drainage system. Which of the following is the priority intervention?

   a. Increase the suction

   b. Clamp the chest tubes

   c. Try to remove the air

   d. Check all connections are secure

77. A patient is admitted to the ICU post esophagectomy. The patient is intubated and sedated. The nurse notes sudden ST depression in lead II. A 12 lead ECG is obtained and is significant for ST elevation in V_1 - V_4 with reciprocal changes in II, III, & aVF. The nurse suspects:

   a. Inferior wall MI

   b. Lateral wall MI

   c. Anterior septal wall MI

   d. Posterior wall MI

78. A 36-year-old female diabetic patient is now 3 days post-operative after a mitral valve repair for infective endocarditis. She is extubated; however, she is developing tachypnea and periods of oxygen desaturation despite therapy with high flow nasal cannula. The CXR reveals bilateral pulmonary infiltrates. The patient is also becoming more hypotensive. Six units of FFP, 4 units of PRBCs and platelets were administered intra-operatively. The RN should suspect which of the following as a differential diagnosis?

    a. Septic pneumonia

    b. Transfusion Related Acute Lung Injury (TRALI)

    c. Transfusion Associated Circulatory Overload (TACO)

    d. Pulmonary edema

79. The Rapid Response Nurse is called to the bedside of a patient who is 7 days post-operative following a right lower lobectomy for lung cancer. The patient began experiencing sudden diaphoresis, light-headedness, nausea and back pain. Vital signs taken by the Rapid Response Nurse on arrival:

HR   58 bpm
BP   78/48 (58) mm Hg
RR   28
SpO_2 94% on 2 L NC
Temp 36.0° C

A 12 lead ECG is obtained and reveals ST segment elevation in II, III, & aVF with reciprocal lead changes in I & aVL. The nurse suspects:

    a. Posterior wall MI

    b. Inferior wall MI

    c. Anterior wall MI

    d. Septal wall MI

80. A patient who received a left ventricular assist device (LVAD) can demonstrate signs of right heart strain when the left ventricle is off loaded by the device and the right ventricle assumes more work. Which of the following symptoms indicate right heart strain?

    a.   Elevated central venous pressure (CVP)

    b.   Elevated pulmonary artery pressure (PAP)

    c.   Elevated pulmonary artery occlusive pressure (PAOP)

    d.   Decreased central venous pressure (CVP)

81. Heart blocks are a potential complication after which of the following procedures?

    a.   Tricuspid Valve Replacement

    b.   Ascending Aortic Aneurysm Repair without valve involvement

    c.   3-vessel CABG

    d.   Aortic Valve Replacement

82. A 53-year-old male is now 4 hours post-operative in the ICU after an aortic valve replacement. He now has right-sided weakness, slurred speech and facial droop. His CT scan reveals a large area of hypodensity in his left middle cerebral artery region. The RN should anticipate which of the following?

    a.   Administration of rtPA 100 mg IV infusion

    b.   Palliative Care Consultation

    c.   Neurological assessments every 4 hours

    d.   Transporting the patient to Interventional Radiology for cerebral thrombectomy

83. Which of the following situations would be a contradiction for early extubation?

    a.   Epinephrine infusing at 0.04 mcg/kg/min with a MAP of 68 and a cardiac index of 2.4 L/min/m^2

    b.   Total bypass time of 120 minutes with the FiO_2 at 35%

    c.   Cardiac index of 1.6 L/min/m^2 with IABP therapy at 1:1, on Dobutamine & 2 vasopressors

    d.   Administration of 2 liters of crystalloid for an arterial pressure of 92/53 (65) mm Hg

84. A patient is admitted to the ICU after bilateral ventricular assist device (BiVAD) placement surgery. The patient is intubated and sedated. Ventilator settings on arrival to the ICU are:

AMV mode

FiO_2 60%

Rate 12 bpm

Vt 450 ml

PEEP +5

The nurse notes a sudden decrease in the oxygen saturation that is not responsive to increases in the FiO_2. Blood tinged secretions are observed via the endotracheal tube (ETT) with suctioning. Patient vital signs are as follows:

HR   110 irregular

MAP 72 mm Hg

RR   12 (set), 32 bpm total

T   36.8° C

SpO_2 86%

$PEtCO_2$ 23 mm Hg

A chest x-ray is obtained and reveals a Westermark sign. An arterial blood gas (ABG) is obtained.

The results are as follows:

pH   7.28

$PaCO_2$ 60

PaO_2 50

HCO_3 24

The nurse suspects:

a. Pulmonary edema

b. Right sided heart failure

c. Cardiac tamponade

d. Pulmonary embolism

85. A patient is on Intra-Aortic Balloon Pump (IABP) therapy for management prior to a planned CABG the next day. Suddenly, the IABP starts alarming, and the RN notices blood in the helium tubing. What would be the issue and what is the appropriate action?

a. No intervention is required, this is normal

b. The balloon catheter has ruptured; immediately stop the IABP and notify the provider

c. The balloon catheter has ruptured the vessel; stop the IABP and notify the provider

d. The balloon catheter has a hole in it but can still function; assess the patient's labs

86. The nurse is caring for a 56-year-old male patient with severe mitral regurgitation, who recently returned from surgery post mitral valve replacement. Within 30 minutes of arrival, he experiences a brief Ventricular Fibrillation episode. The RN believes this was related to R-on-T phenomenon secondary to his epicardial pacing wires delivering an inappropriate electrical stimulus. When interrogating the pacing generator, which of the following should the nurse anticipate finding?

    a.   An over-sensing problem

    b.   An under-sensing problem

    c.   A failure to capture problem

    d.   A failure to fire problem

87. A 70-year-old male with severe mitral regurgitation is transferred to the ICU following a successful, uncomplicated MitraClip procedure. During the initial Pulmonary Artery catheter calibration, you notice the mixed venous pulmonary artery saturation - SvO_2 is 87%. What would be the best explanation for the increased mixed venous oxygenation measurement?

    a.   Left to right intra-cardiac shunting

    b.   These are expected values following a MitraClip procedure

    c.   The pulmonary artery catheter was in the wedge position when the measurements were taken

    d.   Right to left intra-cardiac shunting

8. A patient is admitted to the ICU after a right thoracotomy. The patient remains intubated and sedated and has 2 chest tubes on the right. Tidaling is present in both chest tubes and no bubbling is visualized in the water seal chamber. Patient vital signs on admission are as follows:

HR   80 and regular

BP   122/56 (78) mm Hg

RR   18 (set)

Temp 36.4° C

SpO$_2$ 94%

Chest Tube #1 - 50 ml serosanguinous drainage

Chest tube #2 - 100 ml serosanguinous drainage

Urine output 75 ml

2 hours after admission the nurse is alerted to sudden change in vital signs:

HR   120

BP   90/40 (56)

RR   18 (set)

SpO$_2$ 86%

Chest tube #1 - 10 ml serosanguinous drainage

Chest tube #2 - no drainage

Tidaling is longer visible and vigorous bubbling is noted with respirations in the water seal chamber of chest tube #2. Which order should the nurse anticipate?

a. 2 Liters IV bolus of Lactated Ringers

b. Stat chest x-ray

c. Place the chest tubes x 2 to water seal

d. Clamp the tubing for chest tube #2

89. A nurse responds to a Rapid Response activation on the telemetry floor. The RN called secondary to acute paraplegia noted by her patient, who was 3 days post descending thoracic aneurysm repair. The patient attempted to get out of bed and fell. The patient is complaining of numbness and inability to move her bilateral lower extremities. The RN reports the ACE inhibitor and beta blocker dosages were increased that morning and the patient had a transient period of hypotension with SBP in the 60's, but responded well to a small fluid bolus a few hours ago.

Vital signs currently are: HR 130 BP 88/65 (55), RR 20, SpO$_2$ 96% on room air.

Which of the following interventions are necessary?

a. Call Neurologist and prepare for CT scan of head

b. Administer volume and prepare for lumbar drain placement

c. Give Lasix and hydrocortisone to decrease any spinal swelling

d. Give Glucagon and call the Neurologist

90. A patient with a left ventricular assist device (LVAD) has a hemodynamic profile including: HR 88 bpm, MAP 58 mm Hg and CVP 5 mm Hg. The LVAD alarms "low flow" and the monitor shows short runs of Ventricular Tachycardia. The nurse would anticipate which of the following?

a. Lower the pump speed

b. Increase the pump speed

c. Administer a fluid bolus

d. Administer an antiarrhythmic medication

91. A patient who is 6 hours postoperative from a 3-vessel CABG has mediastinal chest tubes set to -20 cm suction. Once extubated, the patient has been agitated and moving around quite a bit. The nurse notices the patient now has bubbling in the water seal chamber that initially wasn't there.

What should be the initial priority?

a. Sedate or restrain the patient to get them to stop moving

b. Get a new chest drainage system; this one is damaged

c. Check the system tubing connections and insertion site for leakage

d. Turn down the suction; it must be too much

Answers Practice Exam 2

1. C. The inferior wall. The pathologic Q-waves in leads III and aVF demonstrate an infarct pattern in the inferior wall of the left ventricle. Q waves are considered pathologic if the depth is at least ¼ the total height of the R wave, with a width ≥ 0.04. The Troponin-I values may take up to a week to normalize. A cardiac catheterization should be planned for the patient.

2. A. Dosing a maximum of 30 grams per day. Amicar is an anti-fibrinolytic used to control bleeding post-operatively. It inhibits plasminogen binding to fibrin, the conversion of plasminogen to plasmin and then inhibits fibrinolysis. The onset of action is 1 - 2 hours with a 3 - 4 hour duration of action. Initial dosing is 4 - 5 grams IV or PO and then either hourly oral dosing or continuous IV infusion. Administration can continue for 8 hours or until bleeding is controlled, but not to exceed 30 grams/day.

3. B. The balloon inflates during diastole to improve coronary, cerebral and peripheral blood flow. Multiple hemodynamic effects can be seen using intra-aortic balloon counterpulsation in the setting of cardiogenic shock. When the IABP balloon inflates, this can lead to augmented perfusion by displacing blood retrograde to the coronary, cerebral & peripheral vasculature. When the balloon deflates, this can lead to reduced afterload in the aorta and reduced pressure the left ventricle must eject against during systole while the balloon is deflated.

. C. Connect epicardial pacing wires and begin pacing. The priority is to restore cardiac output as the patient is clinically symptomatic with impaired perfusion. Cardiac output is a calculation of stroke volume and heart rate. With a heart rate of 40 bpm, adequate cardiac output is not maintained. Increasing the heart rate will improve cardiac output. The vagus nerve is transected for cardiac transplant and administration of IV atropine will not be effective. Epinephrine could be considered if contractility is also impaired and blood pressure and clinical indicators of cardiac output do not improve with an increase in heart rate.

5. D. Phenylephrine infusion. Phenylephrine is an alpha agonist and promotes peripheral vasoconstriction. The patient is hypotensive with a low SVR, indicating vasodilation. This has an effect on overall hemodynamics having less resistance for the heart to eject against. By initiating Phenylephrine, it will promote vasoconstriction leading to an increase in the blood pressure and SVR without having much effect on the heart rate. If the cardiac output decreases, a positive inotrope like Dobutamine should be considered. The patient has adequate filling pressures, so volume is not indicated.

6. C. Acute Respiratory Distress Syndrome. ARDS is characterized by progressive refractory hypoxemia, bilateral pulmonary infiltrates, and a P/F ratio < 300. This patient's P/F ratio is 68 (PaO_2 divided by the FiO_2 = 68 ÷ 100% = 68) which carries a mortality of > 45% per the Berlin Criteria. Cardiopulmonary bypass was the major risk factor that predisposed the patient to ARDS.

ARDS is managed by protecting the lungs from overstretch by using lower tidal volume & PEEP to improve oxygenation. The goal is to keep the plateau pressure < 30 cm H_2O. This is done by decreasing the tidal volume. In general, "Lung Protective Ventilation" (LPV) starts with a tidal volume of 6 mL/kg and can be decreased to a low of 4 mL/kg. The tidal volume dose is based on gender & height using predicted body weight vs. actual body weight. If the tidal volume were dosed on actual body weight, most patients would experience overstretch of their lung leading to ventilator induced injury.

7. D. Cardiac tamponade. Cardiac tamponade can occur from anything that restricts normal cardiac wall motion and contraction including swelling and bleeding. A pericardial window is a surgical procedure that removes a small portion of the pericardial membrane allowing fluid to drain. Fluid or blood accumulation can develop as a surgical complication and are clinically assessed with jugular venous distention, muffled heart sounds, tachycardia, hypotension, narrow pulse pressure and elevated left and right atrial pressures (because the heart is compressed).

8. D. Prone positioning. Prone positioning reduces pleural pressure on the dorsal lung. This allows for a reduction in atelectasis and results in increased alveolar space for gas exchange and oxygenation.

Albuterol would be a temporary measure and may cause an increase in the heart rate. Although inhaled Epoprostenol (Flolan) is a pulmonary vasodilator, the evidence doesn't demonstrate an improvement in mortality in ARDS management. Nitric oxide may also be delivered by inhalation, but again has never demonstrated improvement in mortality. Steroids have mixed support and are not used as a first line strategy in the management of refractory hypoxemia in ARDS.

9. A. BP 88/70 (76) and CVP 18 mm Hg. Cardiac tamponade is an emergent condition wherein fluid accumulates around the heart and impairs its ability to pump blood.

Three clinical signs: muffled heart tones, jugular vein distension (JVD) and hypotension are known as Beck's triad. It is a collection of three medical signs associated with acute cardiac tamponade. A rapid elevation in central venous pressure (CVP) is often seen, related to JVD.

10. A. Insulin. Epinephrine causes the liver to convert stored glycogen to glucose and release it, raising blood glucose levels. By weaning off the Epinephrine infusion, the blood glucose levels will likely decrease, decreasing Insulin needs.

11. C. Polar, pulseless, pallor, pain. The 6 P's of acute arterial occlusion include: Pallor (pale, delayed cap refill), Polar (cold to touch), Pain located distally, gradually increases in severity), Pulseless (compared to other side), Paresthesia (numbness, tingling sensations) and Paralysis (ischemic nerve dysfunction).

2. A. Hemodynamic instability caused by cardiac tamponade. Cardiac tamponade is an emergent situation that requires immediate intervention or otherwise will result in death. Opening the chest at bedside is the quickest way to relieve the tamponade.

13. C. Bedside re-sternotomy. The patient is experiencing cardiac tamponade. It is a surgical emergency and requires immediate surgical intervention. Opening the chest at the bedside through the previous sternotomy incision is indicated. The goal of this emergent surgical intervention is to control bleeding and alleviate cardiac compression in order to restore normal heart wall motion and function.

14. D. Dobutamine infusion. Dobutamine stimulates beta$_1$ receptors resulting in positive inotropic effects. Additionally, Dobutamine provides some vasodilatory effects. This would assist in lowering the SVR and PAOP, which should lead to an increase in cardiac output. The patient has adequate filling pressures, so fluid would not be indicated.

Epinephrine and Dopamine would be used if the patient was hypotensive in addition to the low cardiac output state. However, both Dopamine and Epinephrine have higher risks of tachycardia and will increase systemic vascular resistance. This may lead to increased myocardial workload & oxygen demand. In states of cardiogenic shock, mechanical assistance, such as intra-aortic balloon counterpulsation or the Impella device should be considered.

15. A. Document the findings and continue to monitor. Safe management and care of pleural chest tubes includes assessment of drainage, tidaling, the presence of an air leak and appropriate suction. Pleural chest tubes do not require stripping. Placing the chest tube to water seal should only be done with a provider order. If the chest tube output continues to be high, the provider should be notified. The slide clamp on the chest tube should always remain open and unclamped to prevent the development of a pleural effusion or pneumothorax and allow drainage.

16. A. Inhaled nitric oxide. The patient is demonstrating signs of right ventricular (RV) dysfunction. Because the LVAD function depends on adequate flow from the right ventricle, patients are monitored closely for signs of right heart failure. Nitric oxide has been shown to improve RV function by selective pulmonary vasodilation, which in turn improves left ventricular filling, cardiac output and systemic arterial pressure. Beta blockers are useful in treating left ventricular failure, but not ideal for right ventricular failure. The Milrinone infusion is required for positive inotropic effects and pulmonary vasodilation. Although the blood pressure is not optimized, the alpha-adrenergic effects of Phenylephrine on the right ventricle may have an overall negative inotropic effect due to increased resistance.

17. D. Open the lumbar drain to decrease cerebral spinal pressure. Hypoperfusion is the main mechanism producing spinal cord ischemia. Therefore, avoiding hypotension, maintaining an adequate MAP and relieving cerebral spinal fluid drainage are important to improve spinal cord perfusion during the post-operative period.

18. A. Calcium. The presence of citrate, an anticoagulant added to banked blood, binds to calcium reducing the plasma calcium concentration. With transfusion of one unit of packed red blood cells, the liver is normally able to clear citrate from the blood. However, with large volume blood transfusion and compromised liver elimination, it accumulates in the blood stream, leaching calcium leading to hypocalcemia.

19. C. Septal rupture. Septal rupture can occur in all types of infarcts, usually within 3 - 5 days after a MI, but can occur within the first 24 hours. Risk factors include wrap around LAD (identified by ST elevation in anterior and inferior leads), RV infarction or large infarcts. Patients present with acute hypotension, right sided heart failure (due to left to right shunt in septum) and a new harsh holosystolic murmur.

20. D. Hemoglobinuria. Pump thrombosis leads to hemolysis and the release of hemoglobin in the urine. The destruction of RBCs causes a decrease in the hemoglobin and hematocrit. Hemolysis releases LDH from RBCs causing increased levels. Heart failure symptoms are a result of poor pump function and an increase in left ventricular end diastolic volume.

21. B. Chest x-ray STAT. A chest x-ray will support the differential diagnosis to support the determination of appropriate follow up interventions. Early mobilization, incentive spirometry, and coughing/deep breathing can help prevent atelectasis. An ABG can be used to determine the degree of gas exchange impairment and whether BiPAP will be an appropriate temporary intervention to support ventilation. The patient likely needs better pain control and aggressive pulmonary toileting.

22. B. Left bundle branch block. A left bundle branch block mimics ST elevation, especially in lead V1. The AHA/ACC guidelines recommend to suspect ischemia in the setting of a new left bundle branch block on a 12 lead ECG in the setting of ACS. Left ventricular hypertrophy, ventricular paced rhythm, resting ST depression, and digoxin therapy also interfere with diagnostic findings and may mimic ischemia on 12 lead ECG.

23. C. Delirium. Approximately 50% of all patients who undergo a TA-TAVR experience delirium post-operatively. The average age of patients enrolled in the original PARTNER trial was 83, and post-operative delirium (POD) was assessed in a retrospective review of the original data. They found 51% of TA-TAVR and 16% of TF-TAVR (trans-femoral TAVR) experienced post-operative delirium (POD). POD is associated with increased mortality, increased incidence of nursing home placement and increased hospital length of stay.

24. A. Stop the Heparin infusion, HIT is suspected. The patient is demonstrating signs of Heparin Induced Thrombocytopenia. HIT may occur between day 2 and day 10 of Heparin administration and exposure. If the platelet count drops by 50% from baseline or a count < 150,000 mm^3 in the setting of Heparin exposure, HIT must be suspected. Clinical signs of HIT include skin lesions at injection sites, petechiae, chills, fever, chest pain and signs of thrombosis including DVT or pulmonary embolus. Patients who experience HIT have a 50% increased risk of developing new thromboembolic events.

25. C. pH 7.39, PaCO$_2$ 48, PaO$_2$ 65, HCO$_3$ 28. Normal compensation would be expected in a patient with COPD and no acute issues. Compensation of the pH would be expected with the pH within normal limits and an elevated of the HCO$_3$. There is no assessment data to raise concern for respiratory distress, changes in ventilation or alterations in homeostasis.

26. C. Decrease the tidal volume to 6 ml/kg. This patient meets criteria for ARDS based on the Berlin definition of moderate ARDS (P/F ratio ≥ 100 and ≤ 200, with a PEEP ≥ 5 cm H$_2$O). This patient's P/F ratio is 141 (85 ÷ 0.6 = 141); therefore, the most appropriate evidenced based treatment is LPV - Lung Protective Ventilation (low tidal volume ventilation), which is defined as 6 ml/kg. These patients are at risk of developing auto-PEEP, therefore compliance & plateau pressures should be monitored closely.

The tidal volume should be dosed to the patient's predicted body weight (PBW), not actual weight. In ARDS, tidal volumes typically start at 6 mL/kg, but can go as low as 4 mL/kg in severe cases of ARDS. PEEP should be utilized to improve oxygenation in conjunction with low tidal volume as a strategy.

27. A. Connects the atrial pacing wire to the RA lead. The atrial electrogram is useful in the diagnosis of SVT and determining between rapid atrial and junctional rhythms. The atrial electrogram is performed on the bedside monitor or with a 12-Lead ECG machine by connecting the epicardial pacing wire directly to the bedside/12-lead electrode using an alligator clip.

28. B. Defibrillation with 200 joules. Defibrillation is the best immediate intervention for witnessed Ventricular Fibrillation. In Vfib, Edison (energy) is the best initial medicine! If the defibrillator is not readily available, CPR should be initiated to support the patient.

For the CSC exam, follow the American Heart (AHA) ACLS Guidelines and NOT the CALS (Cardiac Surgery Advanced Life Support) Guidelines. You may be doing CALS post cardiothoracic surgery, but the exam follows AHA.

Cardioversion is used for unstable tachycardia rhythms. Pacing is utilized for symptomatic bradycardia. An Amiodarone bolus and infusion is often used for Atrial Fibrillation. A bolus of Amiodarone might be given during the resuscitation, but it is not the first intervention.

29. C. 72-year-old male with diabetes. Individuals over 70 and diabetes are both high risk factors for the development of an ischemic stroke after surgery. Patients with Diabetes are 2 - 3 times more likely to develop stroke symptoms due to chronic damage to blood vessels.

30. D. Discontinue any form of heparin and start Argatroban. Thrombocytopenia is common after cardiopulmonary bypass (CPB). Long exposure to CPB circuitry destructs and depletes platelets and requires large systemic dosages of Heparin to prevent thrombus formation. However, a precipitous drop in the platelet count after exposure to Heparin is likely in HIT.

Heparin-induced thrombocytopenia (HIT) is a prothrombic disorder of coagulation caused by platelet-activating, Heparin-dependent antibodies. The platelet activation effect leads to excessive thrombin generation, which evolves into a hypercoagulable state causing both venous and arterial thrombosis. HIT should be considered when the platelet count falls to less than 150,000 mm^3 or greater than 50% of baseline. Management of HIT includes stopping all forms of Heparin and administering direct thrombin inhibitors, such as Argatroban or Bivalirudin to prevent or treat new thrombosis.

31. D. Crepitus along the sternal border and distant heart tones. A pneumomediastinum is a collection of air in the mediastinal space. Though it is rare, it can result from barotrauma and is possible in lungs with poor compliance with the need for increasing PEEP. It is important to follow plateau pressures as well as excessive Auto-PEEP to minimize the risk.

As air collects in the mediastinal space, its most common presenting signs include dyspnea, chest pain and crepitus along the chest, neck and face. Distant heart tones occur as free air collects in the mediastinal space. Chest tube placement is the urgent treatment.

32. A. Assess the blood pressure in the left arm. The endograft may have migrated occluding the left subclavian artery. Additionally, the RN may consider repositioning the arm to see if this helps improve blood flow. The RN should also notify the surgical team as this is a vascular emergency.

33. C. Conversion of the rhythm to sinus and slowing of the ventricular response. Amiodarone is a Class III antiarrhythmic and antianginal. It decreases calcium permeability while increasing potassium permeability resulting in a prolonged repolarization. Often the QT interval will become prolonged with Amiodarone.

In the treatment of Atrial Fibrillation, Amiodarone may be safer than beta blockers and calcium channel blockers for patients with reduced ejection fraction. Amiodarone administration for Atrial Fibrillation begins with a bolus of 150 mg IV over 10 minutes and then a continuous infusion of 1 mg/min for 6 hours, followed by 0.5 mg/min for 18 hours.

Note from Nicole – I know we use Amio all the time for atrial arrythmias, but it is actually off label use. Just a FYI.

34. C. Insulate the atrial wires separate from the ventricular wires to prevent any cross-communication. This helps protect the integrity of the wires, while still having easy access to each set. Securing the wires helps prevent accidental dislodgement and potential micro-shocks to the patient. Gloves should always be worn when handling epicardial wires to prevent micro-shocks as well.

35. D. 60-year-old with liver failure and an initial INR of 2.5. Critically ill patients who are high risk for gastric ulceration should be prophylactically treated with an H2 blocker, PPI or antacid. High risk patients are those with: coagulopathy, mechanically ventilated > 48 hours, history of GI ulceration/bleeding within the past year, traumatic brain injury, traumatic spinal cord injury or burn injury.

Patients who have two or more of the following criteria also meet criteria for GI prophylaxis: ICU stay > 1-week, occult GI bleeding for ≥ 6 days, or glucocorticoid therapy with > 250 mg of hydrocortisone or equivalent. The routine use of PPIs are being questioned for general use in all ICU patients. It is well known there is a higher incidence of hospital acquired pneumonia & C. diff with the use of proton pump inhibitors.

36. C. IV antibiotic therapy for 6 weeks. Management of infective endocarditis includes IV, not oral, antibiotic therapy for up to 6 weeks. Replacement of the infected valve is routine and anticoagulation is not necessary unless the patient has a mechanical valve or Atrial Fibrillation. Patients can present in heart failure and progress to cardiogenic shock.

37. B. Connect the epicardial wires to the pacemaker and emergently VVI pace. The patient's hemodynamics other than HR and blood pressure are adequate. The initial action should be pace the patient to increase the HR. With an increase in HR, the blood pressure will likely quickly recover leading to improved cardiac output.

38. D. Pulsus Paradoxus. Pulsus Paradoxus is an exaggeration of the normal variation in the pulse pressure during the inspiratory phase. The pulse becomes weaker because the stroke volume and cardiac output drop due to intra-thoracic chest pressure changes with breathing. A normal variation is less than 10 mm Hg with breathing. With Pulsus Paradoxus, the drop is abnormal and over 10 mm Hg during inspiration. Pulses Paradoxus can be seen in cardiac tamponade or with a significant decrease in intravascular volume.

Pulsus Alternans is a sign of severe ventricular systolic failure that does not correlate with respiration. Pulsus Bigeminis describes change in the pulse pressure related to the presence of PVCs. Pulsus Variation is something completely made up.

39. B. Begin a Dobutamine infusion. Dobutamine is the most appropriate first step as a positive inotrope is needed to provide improved cardiac contractility and cardiac output. As the cardiac index is below 2 L/min/m², cardiac output and end organ perfusion needs are not being met. The patient will also likely benefit from a diuretic.

Administering fluid would likely worsen pulmonary and right sided congestion and does not support increased contractility. Vasopressors will increase the blood pressure, but not directly improve cardiac output and tissue perfusion and will increase resistance (SVR).

40. B. Desmopressin acetate (DDAVP). General measures to promote hemostasis include rewarming and aggressive treatment of postoperative hypertension. Additionally, pharmacological agents can be used. Desmopressin acetate, the synthetic form of vasopressin, promotes platelet adhesion by increasing the release of von Willebrand factor from platelets and factor VIII from tissue stores. It is also beneficial in patients with disorders that affect platelet function.

Prothrombin complex concentrate only contains vitamin-K dependent clotting factors (II, VII, IX, X) and are reserved for refractory bleeding. Protamine sulfate neutralizes Heparin and may be given if activated partial thromboplastin time is elevated or additional cell saver blood is received, however it may cause anaphylaxis in patients with fish allergies. Phentolamine mesylate is indicated for the prevention or treatment of dermal necrosis and sloughing following intravenous administration or extravasation of a caustic vasoconstrictor agent.

1. A. An increase in the SvO₂. Expected effects of Dobutamine administration include an increase in cardiac output, increased SvO₂, decreased SVR and increased urine output. An increase (d/t improved perfusion) or decrease (d/t vasodilation) in blood pressure and heart rate may also be observed. With the resultant increase in cardiac output, an increase in urine output should be anticipated. Dobutamine useful to decrease afterload when patients cannot tolerate vasodilation and a decrease in SVR would be anticipated.

42. D. Cryoprecipitate. Cryoprecipitate would be a key replacement factor as the patient has a low fibrinogen level. A normal fibrinogen level is 150 – 400 mg/dL. If the patient continues to bleed, an exploratory reoperation may be needed. The patient may also receive FFP or other medications to improve platelet function. PRBCs would be administered for a Hgb < 7 g/dL unless bleeding increases with hemodynamic instability.

Platelets would be considered for a low platelet count. Fresh Frozen Plasma may be considered for continued bleeding despite a normalized coagulation panel. If the bleeding continues and the patient cannot tolerate the volume of FFP, Prothrombin Complex Concentrate (PCC) may be considered. PCC (also known as Factor IX or K-Centra®) contains factors II, IX and X. Some versions also contain factor VII.

43. A. Serum electrolytes. Milrinone may contribute to the development of dysrhythmias and electrolyte imbalances. Specifically, Milrinone can cause hypokalemia and a decrease in the platelet count. Blood glucose levels must be observed closely with continuous Epinephrine infusion, as the patient may develop hyperglycemia. Milrinone does not negatively affect hematocrit or lactate levels.

44. A. Increase the energy (mA). The issue described is failure to capture. Rapid troubleshooting of pacemaker connections & placement should be assessed. When the pacer is not capturing, the initial treatment is to increase the energy (mA). By doing so, hopefully there will be electrical & mechanical capture, which will lead to an increase in blood pressure by increasing stroke volume from increasing the heart rate. Remember: Cardiac output (CO) = HR x SV. In this case the heart rate can be increased to hopefully provide enough perfusion to arouse them to alertness.

45. A. Eisenmenger Syndrome. This syndrome is defined as a triad of pulmonary-cardiovascular communication, pulmonary arterial disease and cyanosis. Eisenmenger's is a diagnosis of exclusion, which all other causes of pulmonary hypertension are ruled out first before a diagnosi of Eisenmenger's can be made. Anemia and pulmonary hypertension are both symptoms of this triad. Many patients with Eisenmenger syndrome have microcytic anemia related to iron deficiency.

Tetralogy of Fallot (TOF) is another cyanotic heart defect condition that is almost always diagnosed at birth or early childhood. TOF is managed with early cardiac repair, typically before the age of 1. The goals of surgery are to relieve the right ventricular outflow obstruction, and completely separate the pulmonary and systemic circulation.

46. A. Dobutamine. A normal SvO_2 is 60 - 75%. Normal RVSWI is 5 - 10 g/m²/beat and normal LVSWI is 50 - 62 gm/m²/beat. When SvO_2 and bilateral SWI are decreased, there are 4 interventions to consider when trying to improve oxygen delivery and end organ perfusion.

These include 1) Increasing cardiac output by using an inotrope like Dobutamine, 2) Improving circulating hemoglobin with packed red blood cells, 3) Improving oxygenation, and 4) Decreasing oxygen consumption with the use of sedation, analgesics or whatever is needed.

Using a vasopressor like Phenylephrine, Vasopressin, or Norepinephrine will only increase the patient's SVR, which may decrease the stroke volume and stroke work index, leading to worsening cardiogenic shock. Using Dobutamine in the setting of low SvO_2 and low stroke work index with adequate filling pressures will provide an increase in the force of contraction, increasing cardiac output and delivery of oxygen to the tissues.

7. A. Prolonged QT interval. Haloperidol (Haldol) can prolong the patient's QT interval, leading to ventricular arrhythmias. Postoperative patients that experience prolonged bypass times, are over the age of 5 or have postoperative complications (i.e. immobility, electrolyte imbalances, prolonged ventilation) are at an increased risk of up to 60% for delirium. Haloperidol is a common course of treatment for patients experiencing hyperactive delirium, characterized by restlessness, agitation, and hallucinations.

48. A. Norepinephrine (Levophed). Severe aortic regurgitation can result in left ventricular volume and pressure overload. Left ventricular hypertrophy and dilation can occur and vasopressor therapy may be required to overcome a vasodilated state immediately post-operative.

49. D. Ventricular Septal Defect. The patient may have a congenital VSD or it may have developed over time. VSDs result in oxygenated blood re-entering the right ventricle from the left during systole. This creates a circuitous flow of blood causing volume overload on the right side of the heart. This further creates elevated right ventricular and pulmonary pressures causing pulmonary hypertension. A holosystolic murmur may be auscultated at the left sternal border due to the abnormal blood flow. Diagnosis is made by Echocardiogram. If the VSD is confirmed, surgical repair would be indicated.

50. D. Place the chest tube to suction. These symptoms are indicative of recurrence of a pneumothorax. Placement to suction is required to allow for lung re-expansion. Although a chest x-ray should be performed to confirm diagnosis of pneumothorax, as an initial intervention it would delay treatment. The patient may further decompensate. Obtaining an arterial blood gas and administering a nebulizer treatment might be indicated, but would not be the first intervention. In patients with a pneumonectomy procedure, the chest tubes should not be placed to suction.

51. C. Acute mitral regurgitation. Large v waves noted on the PAOP waveform can be caused by increased left atrial filling or acute mitral regurgitation due to left ventricular failure. Tricuspid regurgitation and RV failure would be seen on the CVP waveform, not the PAOP waveform.

52. B. STAT head CT Scan with NIH stroke scale assessment. Recognition of early stroke symptoms is vital. The nurse should anticipate an emergent head CT scan order to determine if cerebral bleeding is present. Alteplase is the only approved antifibrinolytic medication for stroke and is a consideration. However, recent major surgery is a relative contraindication for the administration of rtPA and should be considered on a case by case basis. The benefits must outweigh the bleeding risks. Cerebral artery thrombectomy may also be considered in the setting of an embolic stroke. Neurologic assessments will need to be completed after recognition of a neurologic change in condition. A glucose level should be assessed to rule out hypoglycemia.

53. B. Meperidine (Demerol) 25 mg IV push. By controlling the shivering, oxygenation increases and oxygen consumption will decrease. Demerol is effective against postoperative shivering. Increasing FiO_2 will not control shivering which is the cause of increased oxygen consumption. Skin counter-warming or external warm blankets can also be used, but since the SvO_2 is decreased, more aggressive measures should be attempted. Neuromuscular blockade would only be used if all other measures have failed in the setting of an advanced airway & continuous sedation prior to administration.

54. A. Perform a stat capillary glucose. The patient may be demonstrating signs and symptoms of a stroke. However, before that is explored a stat glucose should be performed to quickly rule out hypoglycemia. Symptoms of hypoglycemia may mimic those of a stroke.
　　If it is ruled out, keep in mind aortic stenosis surgery may result in the showering of embolic calcifications. Postoperative anesthesia may result in amnesia, but not word-finding and slurred speech. Naloxone would be administered if the patient were having significant respiratory complications from opioid pain medication. The provider should be notified after the RN has performed a neurological assessment. A head CT scan is likely in the plan of care if hypoglycemia is ruled out and the symptoms do not subside.

55. B. To prevent gastric aspiration into the lungs. The conduit that is surgically created with either the lower portion of the stomach or small intestine lacks the same peristalsis and motility. Therefore, patients are at risk for aspiration. Positioning patients with the HOB less than 30 degrees does not prevent chest tube drainage per se. Diaphragmatic hernia is an uncommon complication from esophagectomy, but is not reduced with HOB elevation.

56. A. Perform an energy threshold to determine the proper energy (mA) setting. Over time, energy requirements (mA) often increase. Since the patient is stable, an energy threshold should be performed to determine the minimum amount of energy needed to capture an electrical & mechanical stimulus. Likely, the mA needs to be increased. By increasing the energy on the pacemaker, the cells will have better depolarization when the pacemaker fires. Because the patient is stable, troubleshooting the pacemaker is the first step.

57. D. Metoprolol. Atrial Flutter and Atrial Fibrillation (A-Fib) occur in up to 30% of patients post open heart surgery. Risk factors include obesity, chronic obstructive pulmonary disease, valve surgery and a history of A-Fib. Preoperative or early postoperative low-dose beta blockers, such as metoprolol, are proven effective at decreasing the incidence of A-Fib by up to 65% and are currently recommended as standard therapy.

Magnesium sulfate is most effective if administered with beta blockers and with low serum magnesium levels. Diltiazem is a calcium channel blocker that may be effective for rate control in A-Fib, but not for prophylaxis. Aspirin is given for graft patency not for A-Fib prophylaxis.

58. A. Increase the atrial mA. Loss of capture for a pacemaker dependent patient requires urgent response. Contributing factors to a loss of capture include changes in myocardial tissue oxygenation and electrolyte abnormalities, fibrin clot on wire tip, or malposition of wires. The first nursing action to ensure capture and proper conductic is to increase the energy or the mA setting. Assessing the sensitivity is important if the pacer is not responding or is over-responding to intrinsic cardiac conduction.

59. C. Aspirin 75 – 100 mg daily and Clopidogrel (Plavix) 75 mg daily.
The current standard as outlined by the American College of Cardiology
(ACC) task force recommended TAVR patients receive Clopidogrel
75 mg daily for 3 – 6 months with Aspirin 75 – 100 mg daily for life.
Patients with chronic Atrial Fibrillation should receive anticoagulation
typically in place of Clopidogrel 75 mg daily. It is also reasonable to
consider anticoagulation with Coumadin if the patient is high risk for
Atrial Fibrillation or valve thrombosis.

60. C. Assess a blood glucose level. Cold and diaphoretic skin is a
clinical symptom of hypoglycemia. Additionally, the patient's increased
sleepiness, nervousness and shakiness are also signs. A neurological
assessment may also be necessary. However, the blood glucose test is
a rapid assessment that should be prioritized especially with Insulin
therapy. The patient may be cold and sleepy postoperatively, but at
this point the majority of the anesthetics should have metabolized
and cleared. Increasing the Dobutamine may increase his cardiac
output and make him less tired and warmer, but should only be done
in a decreased cardiac output state. The glucose should be the first
assessment.

61. D. DDD. When reading the letters of pacemaker BMG codes, it is
necessary to know what the code represents. The first letter describes
the chamber that is paced (A= atrium, V= ventricle, D=dual). The
second letter describes the chamber where intrinsic activity is sensed
A= atrium, V= ventricle, D=dual) and the third letter describes the
pacemaker's response to sensing (I=inhibit, T=trigger, D=dual, O=none).
   A pacemaker in DDD mode paces the atria and ventricle, senses the
atria and ventricle and will inhibit electrical pacing in both chambers
based on the intrinsic sensing.

**62. D. Positive pressure ventilation; when the patient inhales,
the increased pressure creates added pressure on the thoracic
cavity.** The increased intra-thoracic pressure from PEEP can cause
compression of the inferior vena cava, which can decrease venous

return. Decreased venous return can decrease cardiac output, which also has an impact in decreasing the blood pressure.

63. C. Stop the heparin infusion, start Bivalirudin and send labs to confirm HIT diagnosis. The "4 T score" is used to estimate the likelihood of HIT based on clinical data that is easily accessible, while awaiting laboratory confirmation. 4 T scores from 6 - 8 suggest high probability for HIT. When the probability for HIT is high, we assume the patient is HIT positive until proven otherwise. All medications that contain Heparin should be stopped and the patient switched to a non-Heparin-based anticoagulant such as Bivalirudin or Argatroban. Bivalirudin's therapeutic range can be managed by monitoring the DTI (direct thrombin inhibitor) assay and the therapeutic range is 60 - 90 seconds.

64. B. Prepare for pericardiocentesis and/or re-sternotomy. Given the limited visibility and access during a minimally invasive robotic surgery, the posterior part of the heart is not drained effectively and smaller Blake drains are often used, which increases the risk for cardiac tamponade. Common findings of tamponade include equalizing of right (CVP) and left sided pressures (PAOP), Pulsus paradoxus, and low voltage QRS secondary to the heart receiving pressure from all sides.

Decreasing the workload of the heart, decreasing the heart rate, and increasing preload is the immediate priority. Preparation for immediate pericardiocentesis is necessary due to hemodynamic instability. Fluid administration may be a necessary intervention, so the right ventricle does not collapse leading to full cardiac arrest. Increasing the Epinephrine or Vasopressin infusions will only increase afterload, which increases the workload of heart. Increasing Dobutamine increases myocardial contractility and decreases afterload, but in the setting of severe hypotension, it should be avoided.

Bottom line, this is a mechanical issue causing myocardial compression & it needs to be relieved.

65. A. Increased pulmonary vascular resistance (PVR). Elevated pulmonary vascular resistance can be related to chronically elevated left sided pressures, ischemia-reperfusion injury, trauma or injury with harvesting or transplantation, hypothermic cardioplegia, and positive end-expiratory pressure. The transplanted organ is not adapted to high pressure systems physiologically and increased afterload can cause pulmonary hypertension and dilation of the right ventricle. This can cause the ventricle to fail. Early identification & treatment is essential to optimize outcomes.

66. D. Lower the device to 10 cm H_2O and keep open to drain. The drainage depends on gravity and pressure gradients between the CSF and the collection device. As you lower the device with the system open to drain, CSF fluid will drain until the CSF pressure reaches the level at which the drip chamber is set. Raising the device would not allow further drainage or reduce CSF pressure. The device must be lowered to less than 13 cm H_2O and kept open to drain to allow a reduction in pressure and removal of CSF.

67. B. Glycemic control, chlorhexidine bathing, dry sterile dressing. Glucose control with a goal < 180 mg/dL, chlorhexidine bathing pre and post-operative and maintaining a dry sterile dressing that is permeable to air are top priorities. Body hair shaving should be avoided or limited as it increases risks for surgical site infections and hydrogen peroxide and antibiotic ointment to surgical incisions are not evidence-based. They should be avoided.

68. D. Draw stat labs to assess coagulation studies and complete blood count. Several factors put patients at risk for bleeding after cardiac surgery including sequelae from bypass, which may impair coagulation, inadequate reversal of heparin or heparin rebound with rewarming, and postoperative hypertension, which places undue stress on surgical suture lines.

Coagulation studies and complete blood count must be obtained immediately in patients who are bleeding so that more definitive treatment of the bleeding disorder can be initiated. Autotransfusion of shed mediastinal blood should not be used past 6 hours post-op to minimize the risk of infection. Longer duration increases the risk of mediastinitis. Vigorous stripping of chest tubes should be avoided, as this can exacerbate bleeding by excessively increasing intrathoracic pressure.

69. A. Methylene blue IV infusion. Protamine sulfate is the proper reversal agent for Heparin and is often administered to patients after coming off bypass. Overdosing or rapid administration of Protamine sulfate can cause hypotension, cardiovascular collapse, non-cardiogenic pulmonary edema, pulmonary vasoconstriction, and pulmonary hypertension. Protamine sulfate should be avoided in patients with fish allergies & given cautiously with NPH insulin, PCN or Cephalosporins.

Methylene blue can rapidly correct blood pressure with an anaphylaxis response to Protamine. Heparin remains one of the most effective anticoagulants for cardiac bypass, though Argatroban or Bivalirudin can be used for patients who develop Heparin induced thrombocytopenia (HIT) with antibodies to Heparin.

70. C. Cardiac tamponade; call the provider immediately and prepare to suction the chest tubes & possible re-sternotomy. A sudden drop in chest tube drainage, a wider mediastinum than the most recent x-ray, and equalizing PA and CVP pressures indicate a tamponade to the heart. When a patient is bleeding from the chest tubes then suddenly stops, clotting should be suspected. This is an emergency and needs immediate attention.

71. A. Statins. Statin therapy should be initiated and continued in all patients presenting with ACS. Research has demonstrated that statins have anti-inflammatory effects. These effects contribute to reduced risk of death, recurrent MI, stroke and recurrent need for revascularization. Nitrates have not demonstrated improvement on mortality as they are used for symptom relief and vasodilation of collateral coronary circulation. P_2Y_{12} inhibitors and glycoprotein inhibitors are used to prevent platelet aggregation and platelet formation and are beneficial in the reduction for future revascularization, but do not reduce the risk of death, stroke or recurrent MI.

72. C. "There is a risk of changes to your heart rhythm after surgery and it is important to monitor." Conduction system complications are possible after valve replacement surgery. Monitoring for the development of heart blocks and atrial arrhythmias is an important nursing action and priority after surgery. It is important to provide education informing the patient of the risk without creating stress and anxiety.

73. B. Augmented diastolic pressure. Inflation of the intra-aortic balloon during diastole increases the pressure difference between the aorta and the left ventricle. The results of this hemodynamic effect are increased coronary blood flow and myocardial oxygen supply. The augmented diastolic pressure is ideally higher than the patient's unassisted systolic pressure because the balloon is inflated against a closed aortic valve. Inflation of the balloon during this time in the cardiac cycle displaces blood volume into the aortic root (which is where the coronary vessels arise) and into the abdominal aorta.

74. D. Valve expansion after deployment. This procedure requires deploying the new valve structurally near the atrioventricular node. Valve expansion & swelling can lead to interference with the conduction system either transiently in the post-procedure period or in some cases permanently requiring permanent pacemaker placement. Patients undergoing this procedure have significant aortic stenosis, which beta blockade is not indicated, nor typically involves chronic conduction system disease. Ectopic beats can arise from guidewire advancement, not heart block.

75. B. Request a patient care conference to discuss the patient's wishes. Care conferences are an opportunity for nursing, providers, allied health professionals and the patient and family to discuss the patient's wishes and the patient's current state of health. The family's requests may not be congruent with the patient's wishes and/or initial DNR status. A care conference would be an opportunity to discuss the patient's wishes further. Extubating the patient would go against the patient's current code status.

76. D. Check all connections are secure. Chest tubes are placed after open-heart surgery to remove air, blood or fluid from the chest cavity and to reestablish pleural pressure. The water level should tidal - rise and fall slightly with breathing in the water seal chamber. If continuous bubbling is occurring in the water seal chamber, this reflects that air is entering the system and being vented to the water seal chamber. You must assess the system and check tubing for an air leak. Start at insertion site and assess at each connection site for a possible leak and tighten seal as necessary. If this is due to pneumothorax, as the air diminishes from the chest or the lung re-expands, the bubbling should subside.

77. C. Anterior septal wall MI. ST elevation in precordial leads with reciprocal changes in II, III, & aVF is significant for an anterior wall MI. Further risk for lateral wall damage is a concern. Assessment for development of systolic murmurs, signs and symptoms of heart failure, shock and rhythm changes including heart blocks is important.

78. B. Transfusion Related Acute Lung Injury (TRALI). TRALI can occur after open-heart surgery and is usually related to cardiopulmonary bypass or transfusion of blood products. Clinical signs include hypotension, hypoxemia, dyspnea, tachypnea and non-cardiogenic pulmonary edema. Most cases of TRALI resolve within 48 to 96 hours with supportive care.

Septic pneumonia is a potential diagnosis, but would be slower to develop. Her CXR would also demonstrate consolidation in addition to the bilateral pulmonary infiltrates.

TACO is caused by circulatory overload from transfusions. TACO signs and symptoms include pulmonary edema and is treated with diuretics. This patient is developing ARDS.

79. B. Inferior wall MI. An inferior wall MI will present with ST elevation in II, II, aVF & reciprocal changes in I & aVL. Concerns for nausea, vomiting, and risks for heart rhythm changes including second degree block Type I and RV failure. Dysrhythmias are a relatively common complication of inferior wall MIs. Both ventricles are affected by the vagus nerve. When these areas become injured, there is often a strong vagal stimulation which often leads to bradycardia.

80. A. Elevated central venous pressure (CVP). Central venous pressure is an estimate of pressure in the right atrium, which can be elevated post placement. Pulmonary artery pressures typically will be low due to a decrease in right ventricular stroke volume and an increase in tricuspid regurgitation. High pulmonary artery occlusive ("wedge") pressures are indicative of left ventricular failure.

81. D. Aortic Valve Replacement. Due to the position of the valve in relation to the electrical conductivity of the AV node and Bundle of His, heart blocks and arrhythmias are known to occur after an Aortic Valve Replacement.

82. D. Transporting the patient to Interventional Radiology for cerebral thrombectomy. The patient is within the timeframe for a percutaneous thrombectomy intervention to retrieve the clot. The patient is not a candidate for intravenous rtPA (Alteplase) due to recent cardiac surgery and high risk for bleeding. Palliative care may be consulted for supportive care, but is not a priority in the immediate stroke phase. Neurological assessments should be completed more frequently after stroke symptoms.

83. C. Cardiac index of 1.6 L/min/m² with IABP therapy at 1:1, on Dobutamine & 2 vasopressors. Extubating the patient will increase oxygen consumption and potentially drive the CI lower than what is tolerated for the patient. This patient is not hemodynamically stable and does not meet criteria for early extubation. IABP therapy is not a contraindication for extubation.

84. D. Pulmonary embolism. For an intubated patient, refractory hypoxemia is significant diagnostic criteria for PE. Other clinical presentation finds that support a pulmonary embolism include: hemoptysis, crackles, chest pain, increased PA pressure, and PEA arrest. Comparison between PetCO$_2$ and PaCO$_2$ can be useful in the diagnosis of pulmonary embolism. The combination of low CO$_2$ transport and lungs that are poorly perfused but well ventilated (dead space), leads to a decrease in expired CO$_2$ and an increasing difference between arterial and alveolar CO$_2$. This is known as V/Q mismatch.

85. B. The balloon catheter has ruptured; immediately stop the IABP and notify the provider. Anytime there is blood or red/rust colored flakes in the helium tubing, it is a sign of balloon catheter rupture. The IABP should be placed in standby mode. The provider should be notified for stat removal and/or catheter replacement.

86. B. An under-sensing problem. Ventricular Fibrillation episodes related to the R-on-T phenomenon are most often are caused by under-sensing. Sometimes, the R wave may be under-sensed despite a low sensing threshold. This critical complication may have occurred because pacemakers sense R waves by sensing voltage over time. As a result, pacemakers may undersense wide (slower) QRS complexes such as PVCs. Reanalyzing the sensing threshold is essential to fix and prevent further cardiac dysrhythmias. Bottom line, if the pacemaker doesn't sense or "see" ventricular depolarization, a pacing stimulus is delivered with risk of timing during the relative refractory period.

87. A. Left to right intra-cardiac shunting. During the MitraClip procedure a catheter enters the right atrium and a trans-septal puncture occurs to access the left atrium and thus the mitral valve. The mechanically created atrial septal puncture typically closes on its own and does not cause hemodynamic changes. In this case the pulmonary artery saturation is higher than normally expected, suggesting a mixing of oxygenated blood from the left atrium. Shunts can be estimated by cardiac MRI, Doppler echocardiography, or values obtained from Pulmonary Artery catheters, if one is in place. The shunt fraction is calculated by a ratio of pulmonary blood flow to systemic blood flow or Qp/Qs.

88. B. Stat chest x-ray. The nurse suspects a pneumothorax has developed and initial evaluation and determination is appropriate. Bubbling in the water seal chamber is present when air collects such as in a pneumothorax. Fluid administration will not help the immediate hypotension as this may be a tension pneumothorax causing obstructive shock and obstructing outflow of blood from the left ventricle. Correcting the insult is the priority goal. Clamping the chest tube should never be done and could worsen a pneumothorax. The chest tubes must remain to suction and not placed to water seal.

89. B. Administer volume and prepare for lumbar drain placement. Surgery for descending thoracic aneurysm can be prolonged with extensive sequela. Cross clamping of the aorta can result in paraplegia or renal failure. Transient periods of hypotension can lead to spinal cord ischemia. Delayed onset of paraplegia is more common than immediate, secondary to escalation of oral dosing blood pressure medications prior to discharge and subsequent hypotension. If recognized immediately, it can be reversible, but only if SBP is rapidly increased and sustained above 90 mm Hg, high dose steroids are given, and lumbar drain is placed to relieve spinal cord pressure.

If giving volume and placing lumbar drain does not improve the paraplegia, then the damage is typically irreversible. This acute loss of bilateral lower extremity motor function is not related to a stroke, requiring a CT of the head. Giving Lasix just after acute period of hypotension could worsen spinal cord ischemia, and glucagon would only be given in the setting of beta blocker overdose.

90. C. Administer a fluid bolus. The low flow alarm along with the low CVP and marginal MAP indicate volume depletion. In this setting, the ventricle walls will collapse creating a "suck down" effect. This causes irritability in the ventricles leading to arrhythmias and a low flow reading. This is treated by administering volume, not adjusting the pump speed. An antiarrhythmic medication is not indicated as the Ventricular Tachycardia should resolve once volume is administered.

91. C. Check the system tubing connections and insertion site for leakage. Bubbling in the water seal chamber usually means the patient has a break in the system, so all connections should be assessed. Or, it could be a sign of a pneumothorax. The initial action would be to check all connections to ensure they are secure. The patient could have potentially dislodged the chest tube with their movement. If the bubbling does not cease, a stat portable chest radiograph should be performed to assess for a pneumothorax.

References

American Association of Critical Care Nurses. (2017). Caring for patients with cardiovascular disorders: Part 4. *Essentials of Critical Care Orientation* (Version 3.0) [Software]. Retrieved from https://www.aacn.org/education/online-courses/essentials-of-critical-care-orientation-individual-modules?sc_camp=1B0BBE9808C748FEBF0E8A6A0FA91CC9.

American Heart Association Guidelines for Cardiopulmonary Resuscitation and Emergency Cardiovascular Care. (2015). *Part 9: Acute Coronary Syndromes.* Retrieved from: https://eccguidelines.heart.org/index.php/circulation/cpr-ecc-guidelines-2/part-9-acute-coronary-syndromes/

Baird, M.S. (2015). *Manual of Critical Care Nursing: Nursing Interventions and Collaborative Management* (7th ed.). St. Louis, MO: Mosby.

Bavaria J.E., Tommaso C.L., Brindis R.G., Carroll J.D., Deeb G.M., Feldman T.E., Gleason T.G., Horlick E.M., Kavinsky C.J., Kumbhani D.J., Miller D.G., Seals A.A., Shahian D.M., Shemin R.J., Sundt T.M., Thourani V.H. (2018) AATS/ACC/SCAI/STS Expert Consensus Systems of Care Document: Operator and Institutional Recommendations and Requirements for Transcatheter Aortic Valve Replacement. *Journal of the American College of Cardiology*, 25117; DOI:10.1016/j.jacc.2018.07.002.

Bojar, R. M. (2018). *Manual of Perioperative Care in Adult Cardiac Surgery* (5th ed.). Sussex, UK: Wiley-Blackwell.

Boudi, F. (2016). Coronary Artery Atherosclerosis Treatment & Management. *Medscape.* Retrieved from: https://emedicine.medscape.com/article/153647-treatment#showall

Burns, E. (2018). Life in the Fastlane. *Right Ventricular Infarction.* Retrieved from: https://lifeinthefastlane.com/right-ventricular-infarction/

Burns, S.M. (2018). *AACN: Essentials of Critical Care Nursing* (4th ed.). New York, NY: McGraw-Hill Education.

Cohn, L. H. & Adams, D. H. (2018). *Cardiac Surgery in the Adult* (5th ed.). New York, NY: McGraw-Hill Education.

Collazo, S., Graf, N.L. (2017). A System-Based Approach to Improve Outcomes in the Post Esophagectomy Patient. *Seminars in Oncology Nursing, Volume 33* (1), 37-51.

Connolly, MD. Evaluation and Prognosis of Eisenmenger Syndrome. *UpToDate.* Waltham, MA: UpToDate Inc. http://uptodate.com. Accessed January 8, 2018.

Coven, D. (2018). Acute Coronary Syndrome. *Medscape.* Retrieved from: https://emedicine.medscape.com/article/1910735-overview

Daley, B. (2018). *Perioperative Anticoagulant Management.* Retrieved from: https://emedicine.medscape.com/article/285265-overview#a5

Deutschman, C.S. & Neligan, P.J. (2016). *Evidence-Based Practice in Critical Care* (2nd ed.). Philadelphia, PA: Elsevier.

Doyle, MD; et al. Management of Tetralogy of Fallot. *UpToDate*. Waltham, MA: UpToDate Inc. Retrieved from: http://uptodate.com. Accessed January 8, 2018.

Estep, J. D., Trachtenberg, B. H., Loza, L. P., & Bruckner, B. A. (2015). Continuous flow left ventricular assist devices: shared care goals of monitoring and treating patients. *Methodist DeBakey Cardiovascular Journal, 11*(1), 33-44.

Fitzsimons, M. G. (2018). *Management of problems after cardiopulmonary bypass.* Retrieved from https://www.uptodate.com/contents/management-of-problems-after-cardiopulmonary-bypass?search=electrolyte%20imbalances%20following%20cardiac%20surgery&source=search_result&selectedTitle=8~150&usage_type=default&display_rank=8https://www.uptodate.com/contents/management-of-problems-after-cardiopulmonary-bypass?search=electrolyte%20imbalances%20following%20cardiac%20surgery&source=search_result&selectedTitle=8~150&usage_type=default&display_rank=8

Gahart BL, Nazareno AR. (2015). *Intravenous Medications* (31st ed.). St. Louis, MO: Mosby/Elsevier; 2015.

Good, V.S. & Kirkwood, P.L. (2017). *Advanced Critical Care Nursing* (2nd ed.). St. Louis, MO: Elsevier.

Hajjar, L.A., Vincent, J.L., Galas, F.R.B.G., Rhodes, A., Landoni, G. (2017). Vasopressin versus Norepinephrine in Patients with Vasoplegic Shock after Cardiac Surgery: The VANCS Randomized Controlled Trial. *Critical Care Medicine, 126*, 85-93. Retrieved from: http://anesthesiology.pubs.asahq.org/article.aspx?articleid=2587563

Hardin, S. R. & Kaplow, R. (2016). *Cardiac Surgery Essentials for Critical Care Nursing* (2nd ed.).

Burlington, MA: Jones & Bartlett Learning.

Jacobson, C., Marzlin, K., Webner, C. (2014). Coronary Artery Disease Module. *Cardiovascular Nursing Education Associates.*

Kern, M. J., Lim, M. J., & Goldstein, J. A. (2018). *Hemodynamic Rounds: Interpretation of Cardiac Pathophysiology from Pressure Waveform Analysis.* Hoboken, NJ: Wiley-Blackwell.

Kilic, A., Acker, M. A., & Atluri, P. (2015). Dealing with surgical left ventricular assist device complications. *Journal of thoracic disease, 7*(12), 2158-64.

Lo, J., & Hill, C. (2015). Intensive Care Unit Management of Transcatheter Aortic Valve Recipients. *Seminars in Cardiothoracic and Vascular Anesthesia, 19*(2), 95–105.

Lough, M.E. (2015). *Hemodynamic Monitoring: Evolving Technologies and Clinical Practice* (1st ed.). St. Louis, MO: Mosby.

McCuistion, L. E., Vuljoin-Dimaggio, K., Winton, M. B., & Yeager, J. J. (2017). *Pharmacology: A patient-centered nursing process approach* (9th ed.). St. Louis, MO: Elsevier.

Medscape Drug Reference. (2018). Retrieved from https://reference.medscape.com/drugs

Mora Carpio AL, Mora JI. Ventilator Management. [Updated 2018 Sep 8]. In: StatPearls [Internet]. Treasure Island (FL): StatPearls Publishing; 2018 Jan-. Retrieved from: https://www.ncbi.nlm.nih.gov/books/NBK448186/

Morelock, V. (2016). Fluid and electrolyte imbalances following cardiac surgery. In S. R. Hardin & R. Kaplow, *Cardiac Surgery Essentials for Critical-Care Nurses* (2nd ed., pp. 353-382). Burlington, MA: Jones & Bartlett Learning.

Nguyen, T. N., Hu, D., Chen, S. L., Kim, M., & Grines, C. L. (2016). *Management of Complex Cardiovascular Problems* (4th ed.). Malden, MA: Wiley-Blackwell.

Otto CM, Kumbhani DJ, Alexander KP, et al. (2017). ACC expert consensus decision pathway for transcatheter aortic valve replacement in the management of adults with aortic stenosis: a report of the American College of Cardiology Task Force on Clinical Expert Consensus Documents. *Journal of the American College of Cardiology 2017*; 69:1313–46.

Petraszko, T. (2017) Transfusion-related acute lung injury (TRALI). *Canadian Blood Services.* Retrieved from: https://professionaleducation.blood.ca/en/transfusion/publications/transfusion-related-acute-lung-injury-trali

Raina A, Patarroyo-Aponte M. (2018). *Prevention and Treatment of Right Ventricular Failure During Left Ventricular Assist Device Therapy.* 34 (3); 439-452.

Sobel, J. Vartanian, S.M., Gasper, W., Hiramoto, J., Chuter, T.A.M., Reilly, L.M. (2015). Lower Extremity Weakness after Endovascular Repair. *Journal of Vascular Surgery, 61* (3) 623-29.

Starrh, L., Becker, D. (2018). Ventricular Assist Devices: The Basics. *Journal for Nurse Practitioners, Volume 17* (7), 538-544.

Vincent, J-L., Abraham, E., Kochanek, P., Moore, F.A., & Fink, M.P. (2017). *Textbook of Critical Care* (7th ed.). Philadelphia, PA: Elsevier.

Walraven, G. (2016). *Basic Arrhythmias with 12-lead EKGs* (8th ed.). Hoboken, NJ: Pearson Education.

Wiegand, D.L-M. (2016). *AACN: Procedure Manual for Critical Care* (7th ed.). St. Louis, MO: Saunders/Elsevier.

Woods, S.L., Froelicher, E.S.S., Motzer, S.U. & Bridges, E.J. (2010). *Cardiac Nursing* (6th ed.). Philadelphia, PA: Wolters Kluwer/Lippincott, Williams, & Wilkins.

Young Lee, M., Chilakamarri Yeshwant, S., Chava, S., & Lawrence Lustgarten, D. (2015). Mechanisms of Heart Block after Transcatheter Aortic Valve Replacement - Cardiac Anatomy, Clinical Predictors and Mechanical Factors that Contribute to Permanent Pacemaker Implantation. *Arrhythmia & electrophysiology review, 4*(2), 81-5.

Zipes, D. P., Libby, P., Bonow, R. O., Mann, D. L., & Tomaselli, G. F. (2018). *Braunwald's Heart Disease: A Textbook of Cardiovascular Medicine* (11th ed.). New York, NY: Elsevier.

About the author…

Nicole Kupchik has practiced as a Critical Care nurse for over twenty five years. She obtained a Nursing Degree from Purdue University in 1993 and a Master of Nursing from the University of Washington in 2008.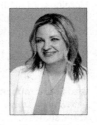

Nicole's nursing career began in the Chicago area. From 1995 to 1998, she journeyed across the United States as a traveling nurse, after which she landed in Seattle. Her first job in Seattle was in the Cardiothoracic Intensive Care Unit at the University of Washington. In 2001, she began working at Harborview Medical Center—a change that spurred an interest in resuscitation.

Shortly thereafter, Nicole was part of a multidisciplinary team that was one of the first in the United States to implement therapeutic hypothermia after cardiac arrest. As part of this effort, Nicole was responsible for protocol development and has published numerous papers & book chapters on this topic.

In 2008, Nicole was part of a team that implemented a formalized Sepsis program at Harborview Medical Center. The program resulted in a reduction in mortality, hospital length of stay and a significant cost avoidance. She collaborated with IT specialists to develop innovative methods to electronically screen hospitalized patients in acute care units for sepsis. For this work, the program was awarded three Patient Safety & Clinical Leadership awards.

In 2002, Nicole obtained certification as a CCRN. She admittedly attended three certification review courses before finally taking the exam! Once she passed the exam she questioned why she hesitated and lacked confidence to sit the exam. Shortly thereafter, Nicole began teaching segments of CCRN certification review courses at her hospital. In 2006, she started co-teaching courses nationally.

Today her courses are well attended and often sell out! Her wit and sense of humor make the course interesting & entertaining. Nicole has a gift of being able to break information down in a way that is really easy to understand. She hopes to instill confidence in attendees that they can do it!

In 2013, Nicole founded Nicole Kupchik Consulting & Education. She frequently teaches CCRN & PCCN as well as CMC & CSC review courses nationally.

OTHER BOOKS BY NICOLE KUPCHIK

Ace the CCRN®: You Can Do It! Study Guide
Ace the CCRN®: You Can Do It! Practice Review Questions
Ace the PCCN®: You Can Do It! Study Guide
Ace the PCCN®: You Can Do It! Practice Review Questions
Ace the CMC®: You Can Do It! Study Guide

Nicole also has online courses available for
the CSC®, CCRN®, PCCN® & CMC® exams!

FOLLOW NICOLE ON SOCIAL MEDIA:

👍 Nicole Kupchik Consulting & Education

📷 @nicolekupchik

▶ YouTube Nicole Kupchik

You Can Do It!

Made in the USA
Middletown, DE
06 August 2024

58626281R00186